# SpringerBriefs in Well-Being and Quality of Life Research

SpringerBriefs in Well-Being and Quality-of-Life Research are concise summaries of cutting-edge research and practical applications across the field of well-being and quality of life research. These compact refereed monographs are under the editorial supervision of an international Advisory Board*. Volumes are 50 to 125 pages (approximately 20,000–70,000 words), with a clear focus. The series covers a range of content from professional to academic such as: snapshots of hot and/or emerging topics, in-depth case studies, and timely reports of state-of-the art analytical techniques. The scope of the series spans the entire field of Well-Being Research and Quality-of-Life Studies, with a view to significantly advance research. The character of the series is international and interdisciplinary and will include research areas such as: health, cross-cultural studies, gender, children, education, work and organizational issues, relationships, job satisfaction, religion, spirituality, ageing from the perspectives of sociology, psychology, philosophy, public health and economics in relation to Well-being and Quality-of-Life research. Volumes in the series may analyze past, present and/or future trends, as well as their determinants and consequences. Both solicited and unsolicited manuscripts are considered for publication in this series. SpringerBriefs in Well-Being and Quality-of-Life Research will be of interest to a wide range of individuals with interest in quality of life studies, including sociologists, psychologists, economists, philosophers, health researchers, as well as practitioners across the social sciences. Briefs will be published as part of Springer's eBook collection, with millions of users worldwide. In addition, Briefs will be available for individual print and electronic purchase. Briefs are characterized by fast, global electronic dissemination, standard publishing contracts, easy-to-use manuscript preparation and formatting guidelines, and expedited production schedules. We aim for publication 8–12 weeks after acceptance.

More information about this series at http://www.springer.com/series/10150

Thomas Jordan

# Quality of Life and Early British Migration

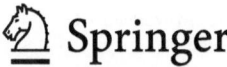 Springer

Thomas Jordan
University of Missouri–St. Louis
St. Louis, Missouri, MO, USA

ISSN 2211-7644          ISSN 2211-7652 (electronic)
SpringerBriefs in Well-Being and Quality of Life Research
ISBN 978-3-030-33076-7          ISBN 978-3-030-33077-4 (eBook)
https://doi.org/10.1007/978-3-030-33077-4

This Springer imprint is published by the registered company Springer Nature Switzerland AG
The registered company address is: Gewerbestrasse 11, 6330 Cham, Switzerland

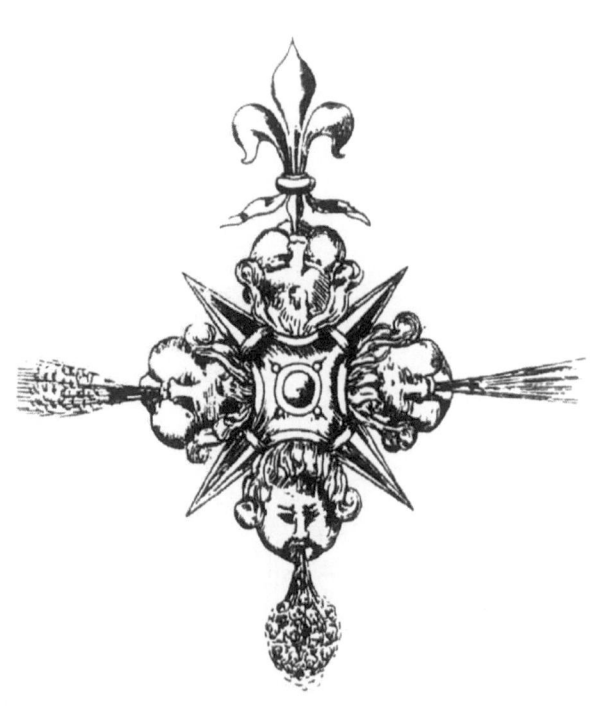

*And having thus endeavored to discharge our duties in this weighty affair ... and to approve our sincerity therein (so far as lay in us) to the consciences of all men; although we know it impossible (in such variety of apprehensions, humours and interests as are in the world) to please all; nor can expect that men of factious, peevish, and perverse spirits should be satisfied with anything that can be done in this kind by any other than themselves: Yet we have good hope, that what is here presented, and hath been ... with great diligence examined... will also be accepted and approved by all sober, peaceable, and truly conscientious...*

Preface (1662), Book of Common Prayer

*O rare Brad Bomanz (1946–2017)*

# Introduction

This monograph begins by addressing elements of this one method in the study of quality of life. Chapter 1 considers ways in which aspects of social life in eras before structure inquiry into the quality of life. Examples are social class, documentary sources on mortality, and ways in which data are set forth. Chapter 2 more explicitly considers an era before our own—the seventeenth century, with attention to estimating the quality of life experienced by British immigrants to the North American colonies. The status and quality of life which people crossing the Atlantic Ocean under the legal contract, the *indenture*, is examined. Their experience travelling to the New World, and their fate there, is appraised stochastically (using the adverb in the etymological sense) drawing on documentary sources.

A second analysis, Chap. 3, describes and numerically estimates the quality of life among Britons condemned to *transportation beyond the seas,* to Australia in the middle decades of the nineteenth century. Migrants include men, women, and boys, and their profiles of quality of life are grouped by gender and by age.

Both groups of migrants are evaluated using a profile of eighteen items, which are estimated using numerical values from −2, through 0, and the highest estimate is +2, to appraise the quality of life. The processes of emigration are placed in the social-political contexts of the seventeenth and nineteenth centuries.

# Contents

# List of Figures

# List of Tables

# Chapter 1
# Quality of Life: Eras and Procedures

**Abstract** This essay applies the concept, *Quality of Life*, to generations before our own, introducing examples from the seventeenth and nineteenth century, and earlier. The gap between the lives of ordinary people and the privileged is illustrated by using examples of index numbers. Data from the seventeenth and nineteenth centuries are presented. Examples of aggregated index numbers provide comparisons over time. Subjectivity as a mode of inquiry is discussed with an innovation presented.

**Keywords** Stochastic · Sir Francis Bacon · NICQL index · Self-worth · *Planter* · Diaries · Death

## 1.1 Introduction

Differences in quality of life across classes have been obvious for generations. When used in the seventeenth century, theatre audiences recognized themselves and the explicit differences in social class. When Shakespeare's Henry V found himself failing in the effort to do more than break holes in the defenses at Agincourt he rallied his weary troops with the well-known cry, "*Once more unto the breach, dear friends, once more!*" He referred to his foot soldiers as a "*band of brothers,*" on the day commemorating the patron saint of cobblers, St. Crispin, 25 October, 1415. But on 26 October, Shakespeare's hero was a brother to his men, no longer. The bond of fellowship connecting Henry (1387–1422) with common soldiers was not sustainable; the social gap between the young man destined to die only a few years later and common soldiers seems improbable despite the flourish of Shakespearian language. On the one hand was the playwright's rich, exhortatory call to arms, and on the other the semi-criminal Ancient Pistol, Corporal Nym, and the other half-starved villains surviving on the hope of plunder and rapine, recognizable to the audience at the Globe Theatre. Prior to embarking for France, Shakespeare's ragged adventurers belonged to a floating population living as best they could, probably engaged in semi-criminal way of life amidst poverty and debilitating outbreaks of viral disease.[1]

Henry's army in France consisted of a small number of the ruling warrior class, and a ragged band for whom a foreign war was preferable to the empoverished way of life which bound their ancestors to the soil. People of Henry V's caste lived distinct from the masses and were connected to the population of England as a source of taxes and as raw material for war's destructive reality. The nasty, short, and brutish lives of ordinary people persisted in that form for centuries after the incident created by the playwright whose characters emerged from the realities of daily life. In this chapter and the next real people will be introduced.[2]

As the mediaeval period slowly yielded to the dynamism of the Tudor and Stuart eras, the barefoot poor remained poor, but some saw in the rise of towns across the British Isles possibilities more promising than the plough and the absolute author- ity of local landowners. Their economic status in the dominant rural society might improve in places such as Norwich and Bristol, and. of course, London. However, the pace of social change remained slow, and towns accrued sub-populations of poor, rootless people. Unwashed, chronically ill, these floating aggregates of unskilled, frequently criminal, individuals were a contrast to semi-skilled and technically pro- ficient workmen who eked out a living. Skilled workers in the woolen trades, for example, lived at risk for fluctuations in trade, for taxes on hearths, and even on windows in the long run. Such levies frequently required funding at short notice. In the uprisings of the 1640s, Dubliners were spared destruction and the erosion of their comparatively good way of life, but their protector, Colonel Henry Jones (1605–1682), firmly levied a monthly charge to support his troops and horses.

In these and other instances we see populations who lived difficult, relatively brief lives if they lived to age five, amidst difficult circumstances which included epidemics and a constant risk for invisible diseases such as tuberculosis and a variety of virus-borne fevers. The common feature for town and country folk was poverty compounded by filth and personal uncleanliness.

And yet they were our antecedents; they ate, drank, and slept; they reproduced and created a genetic and physical heritage which occasionally shows up to our detriment despite the latest innovations in public policy and in health care. Between the pseudo- camaraderie of Shakespeare's band of brothers and today lay generations of people. They constitute a social nexus which informs our understanding of who we are, where we came from, and how our quality of life reached its present level—if only for the fortunate among us. To further our understanding scholars of recent generations have formulated questions of several kinds. An obvious example is the development of biographies of salient individuals in which authors find the well-springs of action, motives, and inner qualities evident in recorded materials. Shakespeare used real

---

[1] In the seventeenth century the disparities of social class were evident to Shakespeare. Later, Samuel Pepys owed his initial appointment at the Navy Office to his cousin, Sir Edward Montague. Their connection began after Pepys completed his education at Magdalene College, Cambridge and he became secretary to Montague. Pepys was always conscious of the social gap between them, refer- ring to Montague as "my Lord".

[2] For an overview of the nineteenth century Irish censuses see Jordan, 1997.

people to fill his literary stage, and presented what he thought were salient passages to dress his characters. On the other hand, groups of people based on ethnicity, religion, and national identity have been treated as a single aggregate in analyses of periods of interest. In the writings of political theorists people in aggregate have been used to explicate a theoretical position. Friedrich Engels used the pitiful condition of cotton workers in Manchester, in the literary footprints of Karl Marx, to explain the failures of nineteenth century capitalism. In the work of those two men we see inquiry addressing an aggregate of individuals who lived at a particular time, in a particular place, whose quality of life they found illustrative of social and economic evils. On a broader scale, inquiry has sought to examine the quality of life of people around the world, and it continues to be a useful tool in many countries. In the early 1990's I surveyed the quality of life for children around the world. The NICQL Index estimated numerically the quality of life for children in 147 countries as the twentieth century drew to a close. Table 1.1 is a slightly abbreviated version of Jordan (1993). Use of the adjective, *estimated*, conveys that reporting information in numerical form does not make such data free from error—note the varying sample sizes. More broadly, among the several modes of inquiry available to investigators the quantitative idiom is conventional, but not automatically more profound or insightful than e.g. personal experience with wholly subjective insights.

However, numerical formats facilitate research and communication among scholars, and follow conventions observed since the opening of the early modern era. Consensus on the value of number for communicating the results of empirical research has its origins in the philosophical observations of Sir Francis Bacon (1561–1626).

**Table 1.1** Mean NICQL[a] indexes estimating conditions of childhood in regions of the world[b]

| Region | 1a[c] | 2a | 3a | 1b[d] | 2b | 3b |
|---|---|---|---|---|---|---|
| World | 67.98 N = 146 | 65.79 N = 147 | 67.81 N = 146 | 70.77 N = 121 | 67.78 N = 102 | 70.05 N = 119 |
| Rich countries | 39.34 N = 52 | 45.58 N = 53 | 38.93 N = 52 | 42.65 N = 43 | 47.61 N = 43 | 42.11 N = 43 |
| Poor countries | 93.16 N = 61 | 82.93 N = 61 | 93.34 N = 61 | 92.36 N = 59 | 82.49 N = 59 | 92.64 N = 59 |
| Africa and Asia | 89.47 N = 81 | 82.89 N = 81 | 89.81 N = 81 | 90.38 N = 70 | 81.21 N = 58 | 90.33 N = 68 |
| Latin America | 51.15 N = 15 | 52.90 N = 15 | 51.12 N = 15 | 49.54 N = 12 | 60.97 N = 12 | 49.43 N = 12 |
| Europe | 30.78 N = 30 | 41.33 N = 30 | 29.62 N = 30 | 32.74 N = 22 | 45.22 N = 18 | 31.44 N = 22 |

[a]The author's National Index of Children's Quality of Life
[b]Author's World Data Set
[c]Includes countries with missing data
[d]Excludes countries with missing data

The first use of the numerical idiom on a large scale appears to be John Graunt's study of a quarter-million deaths, in 1662. In the study of quality of life the need for precision in the selection of pieces of information is paramount. In the case of biological quality of life, height is best measured in metric terms rather than inches, and for weight kilograms are the better choice.

In the British Isles Victorian innovations in the decadal census revealed much that makes their quality of life accessible in a familiar idiom. The result has been a corpus of reports in a uniform style (Jordan, 1998). In particular, the 1841 census of Ireland became comparable to the census in 1851 and 1861. The index Quality of Life for Irish Children (QUALIC) drew on census data in the domains, Education, Housing and Demography in the years before and after the Famine. In Queen Victoria's Irish Soldiers: Quality of Life and Social Origins of the Thin *Green* Line, census social variables illuminate the social context, county by county, affecting the recruitment of Irish lads into Victoria's army (Jordan, 2002).

In 1834, two years after the great reform bill, the Poor Law was amended, a step favoring families in great need. The year 1837 saw innovations in the registration of births and deaths, with the same advancement for Ireland in 1864. Forster's education Act in 1870 was a radical improvement in the lives of children. Changes in public policy often take several years to create noticeable changes in peoples' lives, but the cumulative aggregation of such decadal data across the nineteenth century yields an estimate of quality of life in the era of Queen Victoria. Three such findings, among others, are, The Quality of Life in Victorian Ireland, 1831–1901 (Jordan, 2000); the study drew on fifteen numerical elements in five domains of social indicators. A Weighted Index Quality of Life for Irish Children: 1841, 1851, and 1861. The index Quality of Life for Irish Children (QUALIC) drew on census data in the domains, Education, Housing, and Demography in the years before and after the Famine. In Queen Victoria's Irish Soldiers: Quality of Life and Social Origins of the Thin *Green* Line, Census social variables illuminate the social context, county by county, affecting the recruitment of Irish lads into Victoria's army (Jordan, 2002).

A value of calculated indexes of quality of life is that while conducted for a specific aggregate of data from many domains, e.g., from weather to the price of a commodity such a wheat, is that annual data can be summated to form series over time. There can be annual, five, and ten year time-series, for example, to create a longitudinal view of changes in the quality of life, and to permit a comparative and numerical evaluation of e.g., sequelae to Victorian initiatives in social policy. In Fig. 1.2 we can trace the comparative velocity of change in the VICY index for children from 1820 to 1920. Mitchell's wage index and £GNP per capita show steady improvement across the century. In the case of the cost of living the last decade saw a rise which was followed by a decline. The VICY index increased steadily cross the decades, and increased sharply around 1890. The overall impression is that children's quality of life improved generation by generation. It did so against a backdrop of reforming social policy. Table 1.2 lists nearly a century of policy initiatives between 1832 and 1911. In 1834, two years after the great reform bill of 1832, the effect of social innovations eventually can be identified when indexes of various types are calculated and aggregated over decades. Figure 1.2 presents schematically the course

**Table 1.2** Events in socio-medical progress: Great Britain 1805–1911

| Date | Event | Commentary |
|------|-------|-----------|
| 1805 | Rev. James Whitelaw's *"An Essay on the Population of Dublin"* | A methodologically sound survey of the lives of an urban population |
| 1815 | Patrick Colquhoun's study of the British population | Twenty two groups of occupations e.g. 4.5 million *artisans and skilled Workers* … 1.3 million *farmers* … 3 thousand *royalty and nobility* |
| 1829 | Daniel O'Connell attains Catholic emancipation | Product of the early modernization movement among intellectuals |
| 1832 | Dr. James Kay's monograph on the health of workers in Manchester cotton mills | Pioneering study of the effects of factory life |
| 1834 | "New" Poor Law passed | First of three reform acts widening the franchise |
| 1835 | A. Ure *publishes The Philosophy of Manufactures* | A defence of the factory system e.g. machinery eases the burden of the workers |
| 1837 | Registration of births and deaths | Facilitates study of population data |
| 1845 | Potato crop fails in Ireland | First of several years of failure—grave consequences e.g. emigration |
| 1868 | Torrens Act | Facilitates slum clearance |
| 1890 | W. Booth's *In Darkest England and the Way Out* | Important study advocating training and emigration |
| 1904 | Physical deterioration report | Analysis of health of urban dwellers |
| 1911 | National Insurance Act | Health premiums paid by workers |

of the VICY index against three economic variables. The decline of Williamson's cost of living index became sharp around the year 1900, and the VICY index accelerated around 1890. By using the VICY index and other social factors the consequences of the initiatives in Fig. 1.2 are elucidated over time for the quality of life across the Victorian era.

The origins of innovative ideas are often the work of reformers whose ideas only slowly penetrate inherited social doctrines and values; an obvious example is the reform of factory labor, and mining coal by children, in the early decades of the nineteenth century. Table 1.2 policy initiatives begin with the research of the Manchester reformer James Kay. Sometimes ideas immediately take root, and in other instances the innovator's ideas are too profound to be implemented right away; Kay's work is an example. Reform requires a change in how people think. In the early modern era the process began when Francis Bacon, Lord Verulam, (1561–1626) published his Novum Organum Scientiarum in 1620. In it Bacon set forth the radical view that learning, what we call science, should be based on information developed directly or indirectly through our senses.

Bacon wrote:

> ...philosophy and science may no longer float in the air, But rest on
> the solid foundation of experience...gathered from the facts of nature.[3]

To a degree numerical ideas took root at Gresham College in London, and at Oxford University where John Wilkins lead discussions on ways to advance knowledge. One of the Wadham College group was William Petty (1623–1687), physician and polymath, who asserted that

> By Weight, Measure and Number, God Created All Things. (Jordan, 2007)

In acknowledging Petty's assertion it is worth noting that the elements of Petty's aphorism have a history which can be traced back much farther than the seventeenth century. While it is fashionable to dismiss the Schoolmen of the Middle Ages it is noteworthy that the theologian Peter Reginaldettte, in The Mirror of the Final Retribution (1495), quoted the Book of Wisdom which state that "*All things has God wrought in number, weight, and measure.*" The same statement may be found in the Summa Theologica of Thomas Aquinas.

In our generation, this trend is evident in current emphasis on probability in analysis of numerical data, probability posing its own set of theoretical challenges. They were noted by the poet Fulke Greville in 1633 (Figs. 1.1 and 1.2):

> O False and treacherous Probability
> Enemy of truth, and friend to wickednesse;
> With whose bleare eyes opinion learnes to see,
> Truth's feeble party here, and barrennesse.

Due to his extensive work in Ireland Petty is largely known for his mid-sixteen sixties' survey of Ireland—the Down Survey. In the context of this essay, Petty is noted for his studies in political economy. In 1674, in his Discourse Concerning the Use of Duplicate Proportion, Petty stated that:

> I can produce the accompts of every Man, Woman, and Child
> within a certain parish of above 330 souls; all of which particular
> Ages being cast up, and added together, and the Sum divided by the
> whole Number of Souls, made the quotient between fifteen and 16;
> Which I call (if it be constant or Uniform) the Age of that Parish, or
> Numerical Index of Longaevity there (and) makes a useful Scale of
> Salubrity...such a Scale the King might as easily make for all his Dominions"

In this passage Petty used the terms, ***Numerical*** *Index* and *Scale of* ***Salubrity***, expressions surely antecedent to current thought about quality of life.

---

[3]Bacon's statement was an implicit rejection of Aristotle and the like as the accurate way to understand Creation. Aristotle employed a dualism while Bacon pursued a secular monism. In the seventeenth century critics of the New Learning, as it was called, saw it as the slippery slope leading, via secularism, to probability, and eventually to atheism.

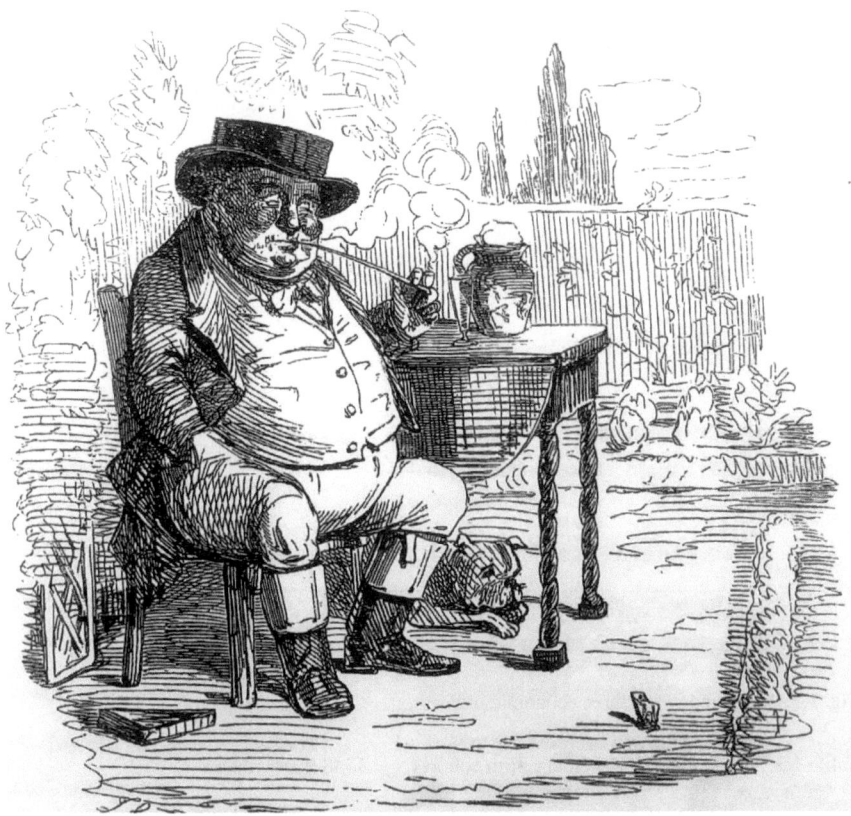

**Fig. 1.1**  John Bull's Victorian self-image

In later decades, two young men in their twenties, from Ireland, John Burn, a bricklayer, and Thomas Rand, a butcher, decided to upgrade their quality of life by sailing for the New World in the ship, *Planter,* headed for Virginia. Those young men and the like are the subjects of inquiry in Part Two of this work. They left no account of their travels, so that apart from their indents (temporary records) on the ship they disappeared. As we will see in Part Two, there is an extant account of life in the New World left by a Scot who crossed the Atlantic in search of a better quality of life. Table 1.4 schematizes elements of life situations potentially influencing the sense of well-being, or subjective quality of life, in men and women across the centuries (Table 1.3).

Table 1.4 is a tentative complex of aspects of life for our own era or those of previous generations. It is a preliminary formulation of factors which shape the achieved self; they interact with a genetic endowment whose vectors of formation are informally encountered. In families traits are sometime observed across generations, e.g., little habits or styles of behaving in family members of different generations.

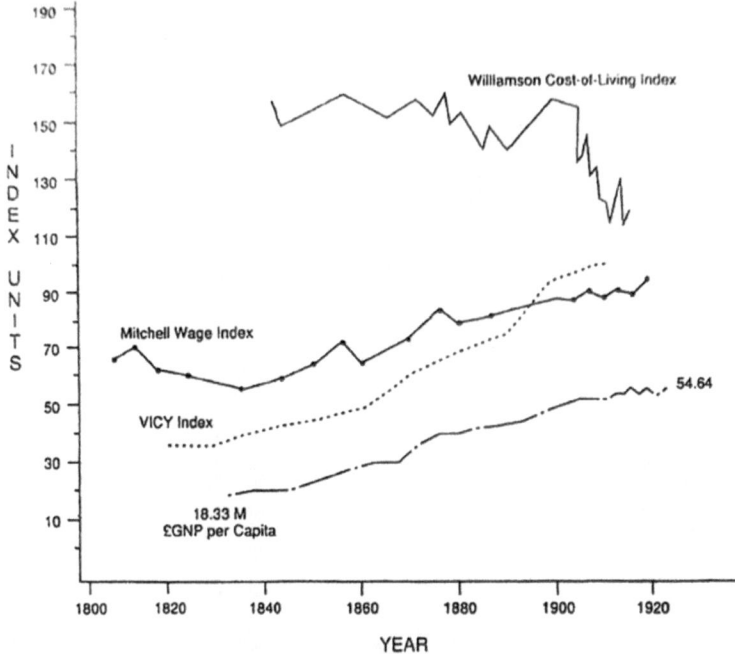

**Fig. 1.2**  VICY index and three economic indicators

**Table 1.3**  Survival in a 17th century birth cohort (N = 1348 live births)

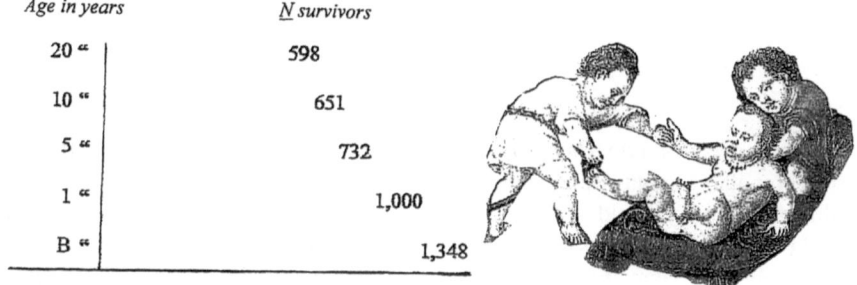

| Age in years | N survivors |
|---|---|
| 20 " | 598 |
| 10 " | 651 |
| 5 " | 732 |
| 1 " | 1,000 |
| B " | 1,348 |

| **Table 1.4** Elements influencing formation of the sense of quality of inner life | Individual | Population | Contextual |
|---|---|---|---|
| | Male/female | Age | Values/religion |
| | Stress level | Marital status/relationship | Urban/rural |
| | Age | Dependents | Social nexus |
| | Health | Census status | Era/date |

A few weeks earlier, on June 15, Pepys wrote in code,

...at noon comes Mr. Creed by chance, and by and by the three young

ladies and very merry were we with our pasty, very well baked; and a

good dish of roasted chickens; pease, lobsters, strawberries. and after

dinner to cards: and about five o'clock By water (sic) down to Greenwich; and

up to the top of the hill, and there played upon the ground at cards.

On the other hand, Pepys' complex quality of life was illustrated by his sexual encounters, in the pattern of the Restoration years. After the death of his young wife Elizabeth, shortly after he closed the first diary, Pepys mourned her loss; he did not marry, but he had a female companion in his life. Documentary sources such as these are rare, and the diary was not deciphered until 1825. John Evelyn's diary is a longer, sober account of his days. The contrast between documents is sharp, but the two men were friends. Evelyn's work, Sylva, was a treatise on trees.[4]

In the case of census data from nineteenth century they generated a number of studies of which an example is, "The quality of life in Victorian Ireland, 1831–1901" (Jordan, 2000), which employed fourteen social indicators to form a time series from 1831 to 1901. The numbers in Table 1.5 were grouped in five domains: *Families =* four variables, *Education and Literacy* = four variables, *Wages* = four variables, *climate* which uses two variables, and *Housing* is one variable. The time series shows progress in quality of life for the population in numerical form.

In contrast to explorations of quality of life from an internal perspective there is recourse to conventional, but not automatically more profound or insightful than e.g. personal experience with wholly subjective insights. Some of the lives examined in Chapters Two and Three are Irish people, and their circumstances were poor. For the 1841 Irish census, Commissioner Thomas Larcom, a military engineer, introduced four classes of housing rising from a level of one for the worst to four for the best. Larcom specified housing quality as:

"...in the lowest or fourth class, were comprised all mud cabins having

only one room – in the third, a better description of a cottage, still built

of mud, but varying from 2 to 4 rooms and windows – in the second, a good

farm house, or in towns, a house having from 5 to 9 rooms and windows –

and in the first, all houses of a better description than the preceding classes."

Given the state of Ireland just a few years before the Famine, Larcom's innovation, while not specifying feet and inches, or the presence of hearths, et cetera, advanced the understanding of quality of living for the population of the four provinces; see Table 1.5. Across the Irish Sea, in Leeds, developers introduced the infamous "back to back" configuration with its limited air circulation and encouragement of the tuberculosis bacillus and other diseases fatal to children and adults.

---

[4]In passing, but only so, the Brief Lives assembled by another Fellow of the Royal Society, John Aubrey, may be touched upon lightly. Aubrey assembled brief biographies of his contemporaries and other notable people. The Lives range from paragraphs to longer passages. Aubrey had one foot in an earlier age—disbelieving almost nothing—but he also was approved by his friends for recording informative anecdotes, and for his interest in Stonehenge.

**Table 1.5**  Elements of the quality of life in Victorian Ireland: 1831–1891

| Variable | 1831 | 1841 | 1851 | 1861 | 1871 | 1881 | 1891 | 1901 |
|---|---|---|---|---|---|---|---|---|
| *Domain: Family* | | | | | | | | |
| Birthrate *per K* | – | 36.07 | – | 24.20 | 28.10 | 24.50 | 23.10 | 22.70 |
| Mortality *per K* | – | 18.10 | 28.95 | 16.50 | 16.40 | 17.50 | 18.40 | 19.60 |
| Persons/family | 5.61 | 5.55 | 5.44 | 5.16 | 5.07 | 5.09 | 5.04 | 5.04 |
| Families (millions) | 1.38 | 1.47 | 1.20 | 1.13 | 1.06 | 0.99 | 0.93 | 0.91 |
| *Domain: Education and Literacy* | | | | | | | | |
| Female illiteracy (%) | – | – | – | – | 35.90 | 26.50 | 20.40 | 15.40 |
| School enrollment (%) | – | 20.00 | 25.00 | 30.00 | 42.10 | 46.50 | 54.10 | 70.80 |
| Attend. ≤ 100 days (%) | – | – | – | 58.50 | 59.50 | 50.20 | 42.80 | 40.60 |
| Letters delivered—millions | – | 24 | 39 | 53 | 66 | 82.24 | 93.20[a] | |
| *Domain: Wages* | | | | | | | | |
| Cork city-laborers | – | 16 | 20 | – | 28 | 30 | 30 | 31 |
| Agriculture | – | 52 | 58 | 86 | 94 | 108 | – | – |
| Masons | 38 | – | 50 | 51 | – | – | – | – |
| Limerick-agriculture | 12 | 14 | 16 | 18 | 21 | 24 | – | – |
| *Domain: Climate* | | | | | | | | |
| Rainfall mm | – | 716.10 | 618.00 | 698.30 | 717.60 | 720.20 | 670.40 | 654.10 |
| Temperature °C (November–March) | – | 6.80 | 6.90 | 5.36 | 5.04 | 3.94 | 4.66 | 5.12 |
| *Domain: Housing* | | | | | | | | |
| N Fourth class houses | – | 491,278 | 135,589 | 89.374 | 156,7411 | 40,665 | 20,617 | 9873 |

[a] 1887

Aggregation of such decadal data across the nineteenth century yields an estimate of quality of life in the era of Queen Victoria. Three such findings, among others, are, The Quality of Life in Victorian Ireland, 1831–1901 (Jordan, 2000); the study drew on fifteen numerical elements in five domains of social indicators.

The study of Victorian era quality of life of people in Ireland is aided greatly by the availability of several summations of social, economic, and other data in the modern era. The VICY index (Victorian Index of Children and Youth) is indexed to the conditions of life prior to the war of 1914–1918. It employs twelve variables in the four domains: *Health* = four variables, *Economics* = four variables, *Social* = three variables, *Housing* = one variable (Jordan, 1992).

Figure 1.2 illustrated the course of the quality of life of children in an era of rising economic growth. Before the criterion year, the course of children's quality of life began badly in the early nineteenth century. Children worked underground in coal mines and were employed in factories under harsh conditions, but they began a slow climb towards decency with schools and reforming laws. The conscience of the Victorian public was aroused by the reports of the factory inspectors, and the excellent propaganda of the advocates for relieving the abuses endured by children. To convey the process of social improvement more concretely than relying on index numbers Table 1.5 presents five aspects of Victorian life. Table 1.6 lists a century of change in items ranging from population growth in Manchester to the price of a four pound (lb.) loaf.

A narrower focus is evident when we consider data to study quality of life at the local level. Dublin provides an interesting example of an error which turned out

**Table 1.6** Victorian Britain and conditions of life: social and economic trends

| Year | Population Manchester (000)[a] | $\underline{N}$ persons per family[b] | Rousseau price index[a] | 4.3 lb. loaf price in pennies[a] | Mortality all ages per (000)[a] |
|---|---|---|---|---|---|
| 1801 | 75 | 4.69 | 188 | 15.50 | 24.7[c] |
| 1811 | 89 | 4.74 | 178 | 14.00 | 24.30[c] |
| 1821 | 126 | 4.81 | 121 | 9.50 | 24.10[c] |
| 1831 | 182 | 4.71 | 112 | 10.00 | 30.20 |
| 1841 | 235 | 4.80[c] | 121 | 9.00 | 21.60 |
| 1851 | 303 | 4.83 | 91 | 6.75 | 22.00 |
| 1861 | 339 | 4.47 | 115 | 9.00 | 21.60 |
| 1871 | 351 | 4.50 | 115 | 9.00 | 22.60 |
| 1881 | 462 | 4.61 | 99 | 7.04 | 18.90 |
| 1891 | 505 | 4.73 | 86 | 6.21 | 19.00 |
| 1901 | 544 | 4.62 | 86 | 5.00 | 16.90 |
| 1911 | 714 | – | 102 | 5.50 | 14.60 |

[a]Mitchell and Deane (1971). See Engels (1845)
[b]Cook and Keith (1975)
[c]Estimated

well. In the case of seventeenth century Dublin the normal course would have been for the officers of a parish Vestry to send parish secular records for storage in a city facility. In the case of records from Dublin's approximately fourteen parishes the legal prescription routinely was not followed. Had the materials gone to the central office they would have been destroyed in the chaos of the civil war of 1922. In the case of Dublin's parish archives a set of seventeenth century parish records was found, in the *nineteenth* century, at an informal market. The small document lay on a blanket, but it was found there by a perceptive passer-by who retrieved it (Figs. 1.3 and 1.4).

Much of the vestries' business was routine, maintaining the fabric of the churches, but they also met the legal requirement to report deaths, and whatever fatal condition the Searchers could ascertain from their required visits to the site of the death (Jordan, 2017). Figure 1.5 is a woodcut of a funeral procession. Beneficiaries of the vestry's charity were orphans who were placed with parishioners who received a fee—usually continued after demonstrating that the child was thriving—an aspect of quality of life. Death was no respecter of social position:

Sir Robert Cotton lost this year 5 daughters which was then
all the children he then had in three days time. (Illick, 1975)

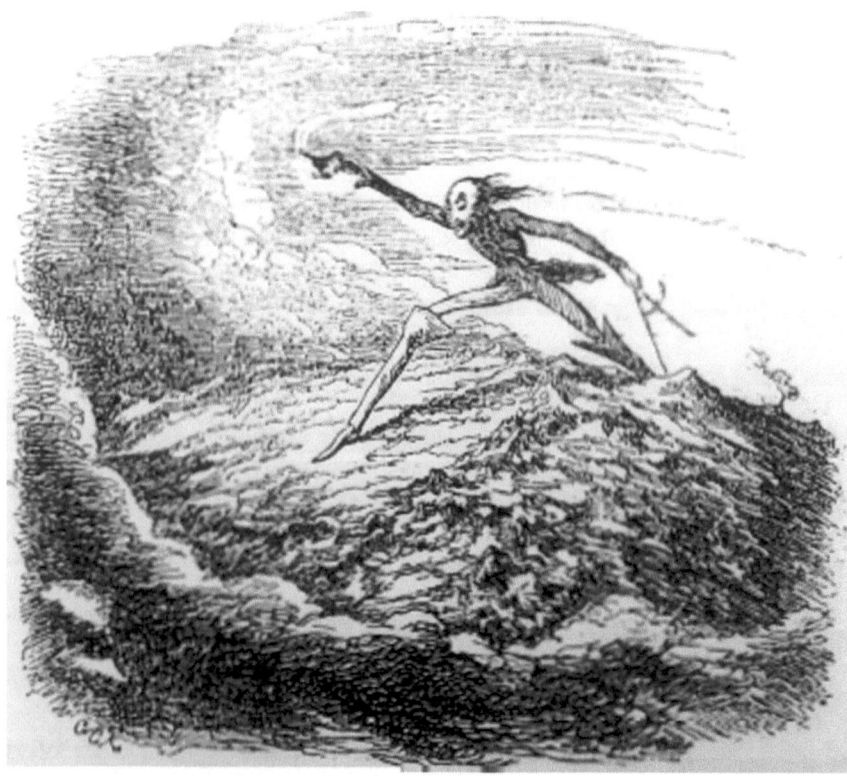

**Fig. 1.3** "Science making giant strides"

**Fig. 1.4**   Queen Victoria and
Prince Albert (*c*.1850)

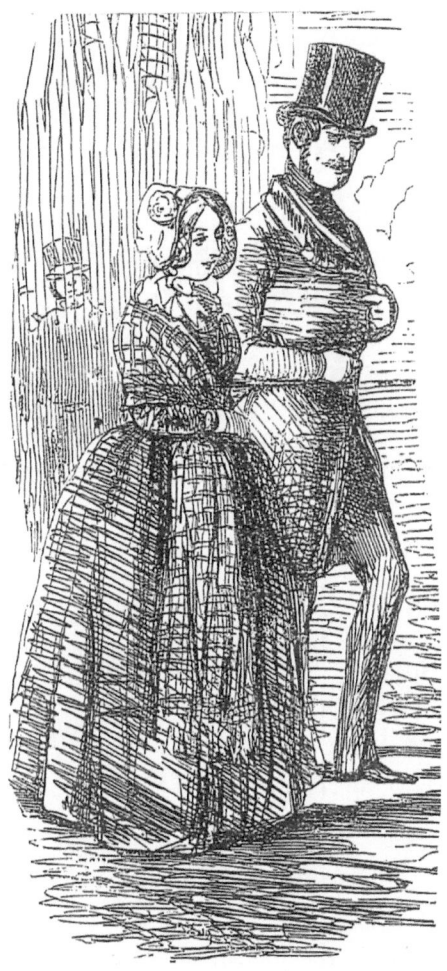

Figure 1.6 indicates that the mortality rate was highest among babies, and that the
rate for survival declined rapidly at ages which we live vigorously. A majority in a
birth cohort died in the first decade of life, and half were gone by age thirty. Figure 7
is a seventeenth century illustration of a burial procession. Leading the group are two
women appointed by a parish Vestry to act as Searchers. In that capacity they were
dispatched by the Register to visit the site of the death, and ascertain the cause of
death. The Register walks behind ringing a hand bell, followed by members of the
parish Vestry. This is a civil rather than a religious occasion, and the person interred
probably was a charity case.

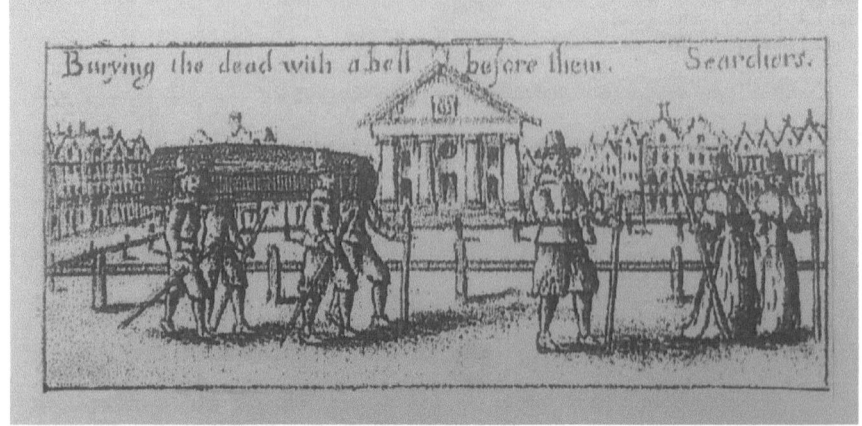

**Fig. 1.5** A burial procession led by Searchers and the Register (sic)

| 50 | " | | 346 |
| 40 | " | | 445 |
| 30 | " | | 531 |
| 20 | " | | 598 |
| 10 | " | | 651 |
| 5 | " | | 732 |
| 1 | " | | 1,000 |
| B. | " | | 1,348 |

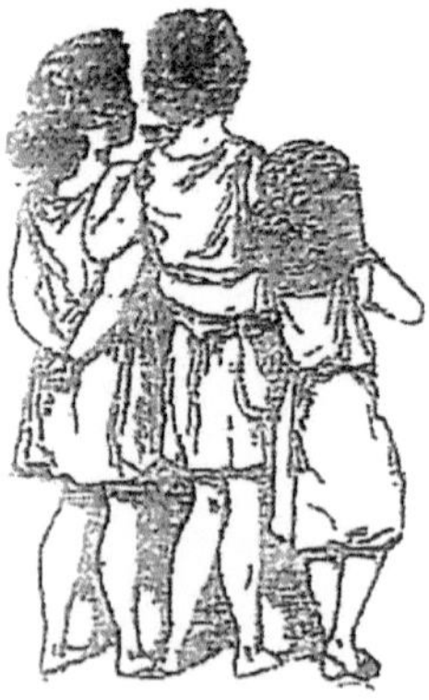

**Fig. 1.6** 17th century survivorship to age fifty

Beyond the antibiotics which contribute to health today is the complex of personal and social elements of cleanliness. Personal hygiene is a fairly recent arrival in the social history of mankind. Samuel Pepys, William Petty, and the Fellows of the Royal Society, rarely bathed.

It is possible that smallpox killed the two little children of Sir William Petty, one of whom was a *chrisom*—too young to have been baptized and named. The Pettys had three more children, and the family heritage was perpetuated in Ireland through their daughter, Anne. The male line extinguished at the death of a grandson.

Conventionally, quality of life draws on aggregates of annual social indicators. Their numerical form projects a degree of objectivity which is partially accurate. In the case of children's quality of life the Irish and British versions employ several domains of information. However, the several versions are used for the entire nineteenth century; on closer inspection it appears that, for children in Manchester, Birmingham, and Leeds the early decades were, in fact, shaped by abuses in the factory system. In the later decades, especially after 1870, education was the prevailing influence. Ideally, the later decades would have drawn on academic achievement data. Such information is not available in aggregated form and, for the earliest decades data on schooling are insufficient. For children in Ireland, over the same decades, factory work was less likely in a largely rural economy. Data on the prevalence of English, as contrasted with Gaelic, would have been useful in developing an index of quality of life. Accordingly, seemingly accurate indexes of quality of life for children are not without their limitations. Procedurally, a subjective adjustment created an array of domains from which the indices were formed; that is to say *subjectivity* in the choice of domains from the set of extant domains is not wholly absent.

In the approach to an interesting set of people in the tumultuous seventeenth century, English—speaking men and women who sought an improved quality of life in the colonies of America's eastern coast, I developed a way to enhance a subjective appraisal of their lives before, during,

Another method of evaluating the condition of emigrants is given in the Appendix. It is a hypothetical estimate of emigration in general for the several groups of people treated in this work. The Appendix addresses no particular group of emigrants, and lists eighteen elements of quality of life for which a five-point estimate is possible, ranging from a negative $-2$, through a zero (a question mark implying irrelevance/ambiguity), and up to a positive $+2$. Sets of estimates are verbalized in the following two chapters which address specific populations—free immigrants, convicts, male and female convicts, and male juvenile convicts.

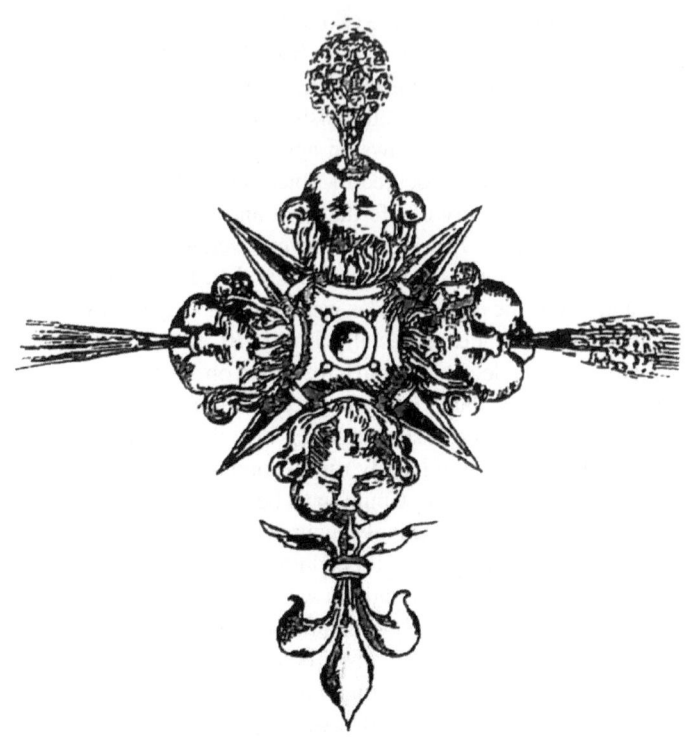

## Appendix: An Estimate of Emigrants' Quality of Life

| Domain | Rating | | | | |
|---|---|---|---|---|---|
| | −2 | −1 | 0 | +1 | +2 |
| Gender (M) | | | | | ☺ |
| Skills | | | | ☺ | |
| Single | | | | | ☺ |
| Convicted | ☹ | | | | |
| Assets | | | | | ☺ |
| English-speaking | | | | | ☺ |
| Prior health | | ☹ | | | |
| Nearby port | | | | ☺ | |
| New climate | | | ? | | |
| Food at hand | | | | | ☺ |

(continued)

(continued)

| Domain | Rating | | | | |
|---|---|---|---|---|---|
| | *−2* | *−1* | *0* | *+1* | *+2* |
| Barber/surgeon | | | | ☺ | |
| Sturdy vessel | | | | | ☺ |
| Kith and kin | | | | | ☺ |
| Property | | | | ☺ | |
| Urban settlement | | | | | ☺ |
| Indenture—*Discharged* | | | | | ☺ |
| − *Cheated* | ☹ | | | | |
| − *Fled* | ☹ | | | | |

# References

Cook, C., & Keith, B. (1975). *British historical facts 1839–1900*. New York: Macmillan.

Engels, F. (1845). *The condition of the working class in England*. Moscow: Progress.

Illick, J. (1975). Child rearing in seventeenth century England and America. In L. de Mause (Ed.), *The history of childhood*. New York: Harper.

Jordan, T. E. (1992). *An imaginative empiricist: Thomas Aiskew larcom (1800–1879) and Victorian Ireland*. Lewiston, NY: Mellen.

Jordan, T. E. (1993). Estimating the quality of life for children around the world: NICQL—92. *Social Indicators Research, 30*, 17–38.

Jordan, T. E. (1998). *The census of Ireland 1821–1911*. General reports. Three volumes. Lewiston, NY: Mellen.

Jordan, T. E. (2000). The quality of life in Victorian Ireland. 1831–1911. *New Hibernia Review, 4*, 103–121.

Jordan, T. E. (2002). Queen Victoria's Irish soldiers; quality of life and social origins of the *green line*. *Social Indicators Research, 57*, 73–78.

Jordan, T. E. (2007). *A copper farthing: Sir William Petty (1623–1687) and his times*. Sunderland (UK) University of Sunderland Press.

Jordan, T. E. (2017). *Quality of life and mortality in seventeenth century London and Dublin*. New York: Springer.

Mitchell, B. R., & Deane, P. (1962). *Abstract of british historical statistics*. Cambridge: Cambridge University Press.

# Chapter 2
# Seventeenth Century Immigrants to North America

**Abstract** For an essay on quality of immigrant life in the age of sail objective data are rare. Here, a process of estimation is enhanced, and qualified, using stages of the emigration process. Two journals of the era, those of Scots, Janet Schaw, and John Harrower, provide a personal link to events in the three-stage model of the experiences of travelers, many of whom were indentured servants. With the information from the Scots' journals and a stochastic model of emigration we come a little closer to understanding the quality of life experienced by vital, energetic people seeking a higher quality of life across the Atlantic, in the age of sail.

**Keywords** Immigrant · Chesapeake · Indenture · Janet Schaw · John harrower · Redemption

## 2.1 Introduction

The environment in which the subjects of this essay pondered their circumstances and the possibilities for their respective futures may be described in several ways. Geographically, they lived on a set of islands once joined to the soil of France, a separation which, in geological time, is a fairly recent event. Within the geographic idiom, they lived on several regions, the largest of which we know as England and Wales, and Scotland; Smaller and to the west lies Ireland, the most westerly point of the Eurasian land mass. Ireland combines a central bowl of nourishing soil within a partial rim of more rugged land. West of Scotland, and to the north, are comparatively small islands whose inhabitants carved out a living in the presence of wind and rain, and from soil exhausted by natural forces. The entirety we know as the British Isles, and its peoples in the early modern era are the subject of this inquiry. Within that broad grouping many individuals lived in the pattern of their forebears—farming, engaging in small manufactures, and trading. domestically; they traded broadly in the geographic world as the limitations of commerce and sea-born technology permitted. However, the rewards for leaving the ancestral village which were a theme in the local environment reached a peak in the nineteenth century (Jordan, 1993a, 2013) (Fig. 2.1).

T. Jordan, *Quality of Life and Early British Migration*,
SpringerBriefs in Well-Being and Quality of Life Research,
https://doi.org/10.1007/978-3-030-33077-4_2

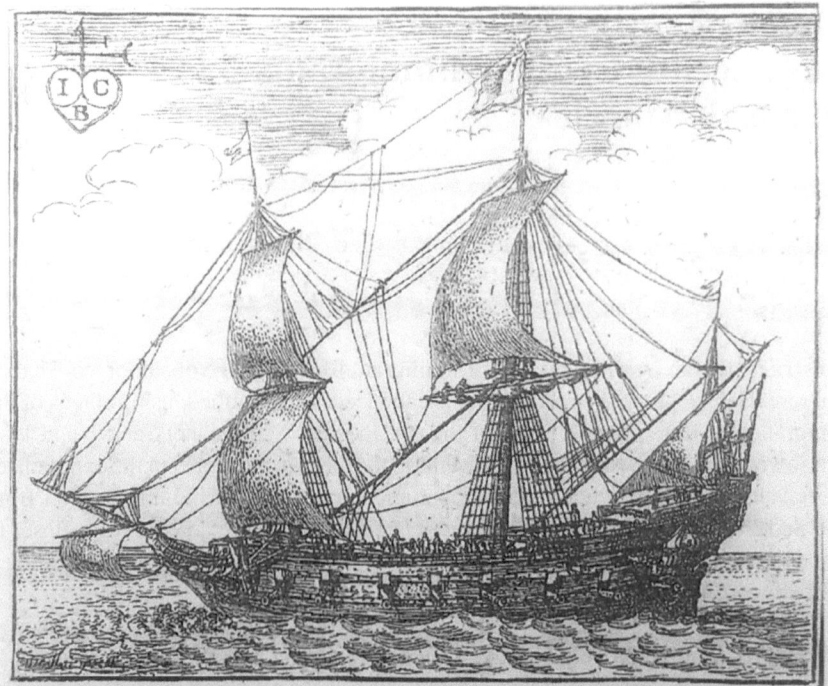

**Fig. 2.1** Indentured servants venturing from Bristol to Annapolis

The several societies in the Britain of the early modern era consisted of villages and small towns spread from Land's End in the southwest, connoting the challenges and opportunities from the counties of Wessex to Peterhead and the Shetlands in northern Scotland, the latter settlements with genetic ties to Scandinavian ancestors.

While the population of Britain was small, its elements permit some cautious generalities. Politically, there were major components under kings; the Stuarts and descendants influenced the major geographic sites, viz. *James I* and *VI*, whose sons and grandson presided over the nation with differing degrees of success. One of them, Charles II, established the Royal Society whose luminaries broke new ground in the form of scientific inquiries. Our world was ushered into the modern era through the contributions of Isaac Newton, Christopher Wren, Robert Hooke, and William Petty. The group convened in 1662 as the Royal Society for the Advancement of Natural Knowledge, with Charles I as patron.

However, the common man, in his cottage far from such eminent scientists, coped with the threats to his modest quality of life as best he and his family could. For sickness there were herbal and alcohol-based remedies and little more. Babies died by the score (see Fig. 1.3), and remedies for animal diseases were largely unknown. People knew a little of the world beyond the immediate environs, and others had ventured to Norwich, Bristol, and Dublin. Some returned with vivid memories of busy streets, large churches, and exotic displays such as elephants, tigers, and monkeys. Some did not live to report the visual riches they had encountered; the urban areas had their own local versions of viruses to which visitors had not acquired immunity. Visitors took back to their communities' strains of diseases which spread by personal contact.

For the sickened, the intimacy of life in crowded circumstances created fear, and the number of the sick strained a sense of obligation to assist. Small communities lived by conventions which included the corporal morality of caring for the sick and disabled. The vestry of the local church, led by the Minister, gave assistance to the needy, most of whom would be neighbors.

Conventions in church attendance, morality, and honesty were fully entrenched in the substance of daily life. The virtues were preached and their breach was scorned. The manor house expected the farmers' rent on time, if only to pay for converting a modest structure into a landscaped country house, and the minister noted absences from church services. The result was a restricted way of life unquestioned by most, but a burden to some.

But the great magnet was the city which attracted people from all over to London. Sited in the comparatively mild climate of southeast England the population of the metropolis was annually decimated by communicable diseases, a demographic trauma which, statistics tell us, was remedied within a few years as immigrants headed for the bright lights. In London, the Globe Theatre with its presentation of Shakespeare's Henry V and the comedies, enthralled country bumpkins. The many entertainments and the innovation of coffee houses, where refreshment could be combined with commerce; and ale-houses delighted the rank and file. Indeed, the prospect was so inviting that some would-be emigrants decided that London had all that one might wish for, and looked for work. In such a setting there were openings for the skilled trades, but for the unskilled, opportunities were fewer. London had a floating population who were uncertain about their next meal, and where they would sleep that night.

In Bailyn's (1985) study of English emigrants he identified twenty three occupational groups among 6190 emigrants. Each of those groups was an aggregation of emigrants' self-reports, titles which were seemingly endless in specificity. Their accuracy was not assured, and some indentured servants claimed more skill and occupational status than they actually had. Never the less, London absorbed them, and the great city became either a staging area before emigrating or they simply disappeared into the Five Points slum and similar districts. The metropolitan area had a floating population of poor and unskilled men and women whose disorganized lives presented a challenge to survival. Crime was widespread, and streets teemed with cut-purses and tricksters of all kinds. A trick for women was to sign on as a housemaid, and then abscond with the clothing provided. Samuel Pepys' young wife Elizabeth was the victim of such trickery.

On the other hand, there were fortunes to be made by trickery or diligence in the streets of the City, the business center known by that name today. Of course, the population included saintly people. Quakers, in their early days, were occasionally violent, and they were disliked. Sometimes, an evangelist, like Solomon Eagle, would parade through the streets proclaiming the end was nigh. In the person of James Venner and the Fifth Monarchists, religious conviction burst into an uprising which was quickly suppressed. Restoration government was composed of men with tolerance for many things; but law, order, and convention must prevail.

In the early modem era there were two frontiers challenging the desperate and the ambitious in the British Isles. The first was Ireland, and beyond lay the distant shores of a continent—North America. The second frontier was the arc of sparse settlements from Nova Scotia, through the Chesapeake region and the territories known at one time, respectively, as East and West Florida, ending in the British West Indies (Fig. 2.2, Table 2.1).

To consider migrating to North America required a shift of imagination comparable to contemplating settlements on the planet Mars, today. From Land's End to John O'Groats awareness that emigration might raise one's quality of life entered the sensibilities of the age. Around the periphery, the Scottish crofter and wife glimpsed a better life for their bairns; they heard of localities where their accent and the local

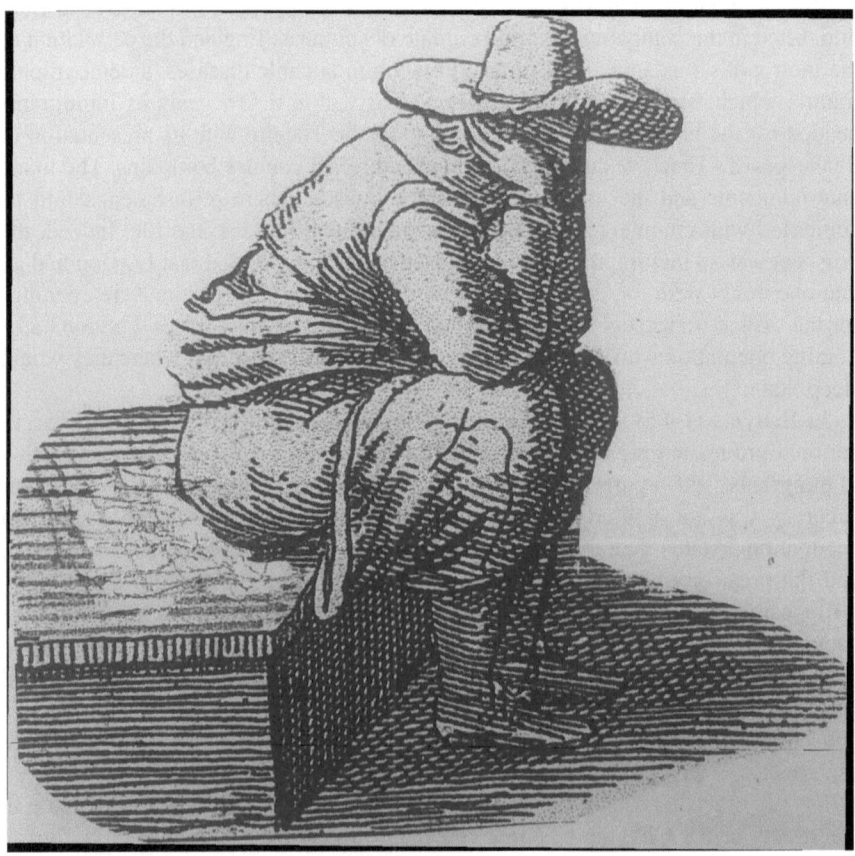

**Fig. 2.2** "Stay and starve—or, go and prosper?"

**Table 2.1** London's annual bill of mortality: 1665

## 1665.

### A General BILL for this present Year,

Ending the 19th Day of December: 1665.

According to the Report made to the King's most excellent Majesty,

By the Company of Parish Clerks of LONDON, &c.

|  | Bur. | Pla. |  | Bur. | Pla. |
|---|---|---|---|---|---|
| ALBAN Wood-street | 200 | 121 | St Helen's | 108 | 75 |
| Alhallows Barking | 514 | 330 | St James Dukes Place | 262 | 190 |
| Alhallows Bread-street | 65 | 16 | St James Garlickhithe | 189 | 118 |
| Alhallows Great | 455 | 426 | St John Baptist | 138 | 83 |
| Alhallows Honey-lane | 10 | 5 | St John Evangelist | 9 | 0 |
| Alhallows Lesse | 399 | 175 | St John Zachary | 85 | 54 |
| Alhallows Lombard-street | 90 | 62 | St Katherine Coleman | 299 | 213 |
| Alhallows Staining | 185 | 112 | St Katherine Creechurch | 335 | 231 |
| Alhallows the Wall | 500 | 356 | St Lawrence Jewry | 94 | 48 |
| St Alphage | 271 | 115 | St Lawrence Pountney | 214 | 140 |
| St Andrew Hubbard | 71 | 42 | St Leonard Fofter-lane | 335 | 215 |
| St Andrew Undershaft | 274 | 189 | St Leonard Eastcheap | 103 | 43 |
| St Andrew Wardrobe | 476 | 308 | St Magnus Parifh | 103 | 66 |
| St Ann Aldersgate | 282 | 197 | St Margaret Lothbury | 100 | 66 |
| St Ann Black Friars | 652 | 467 | St Margaret Moses | 38 | 25 |
| St Antholin's Parifh | 58 | 33 | St Margaret New Fifh-street | 114 | 66 |
| St Auftin's Parifh | 43 | 20 | St Margaret Patons | 49 | 24 |
| St Bartholomew Exchange | 73 | 51 | St Mary Abchurch | 99 | 54 |
| St Bennet Fink | 47 | 22 | St Mary Aldermanbury | 181 | 109 |
| St Bennet Gracechurch | 57 | 41 | St Mary Aldermary | 105 | 75 |
| St Bennet Paul's Wharf | 358 | 171 | St Mary le Bow | 64 | 36 |
| St Bennet Sherehog | 11 | 1 | St Mary Bothaw | 55 | 30 |
| St Botolph Billingfgate | 83 | 50 | St Mary Colechurch | 17 | 6 |
| Chrift Church | 653 | 467 | St Mary Hill | 94 | 64 |
| St Chriftopher | 60 | 47 | St Mary Mounthaw | 54 | 37 |
| St Clement Eaftcheap | 88 | 20 | St Mary Somerfet | 342 | 262 |
| St Dionis Backchurch | 78 | 27 | St Mary Staining | 47 | 27 |
| St Dunftan Eaft | 265 | 150 | St Mary Woolchurch | 65 | 33 |
| St Edmund Lombard-ftreet | 70 | 86 | St Mary Woolnoth | 75 | 38 |
| St Ethelborough | 595 | 105 | St Martin Ironmonger-lane | 21 | 11 |
| St Faith's | 104 | 70 | St Martin Ludgate | 196 | 128 |
| St Fofter's | 144 | 105 | St Martin Orgars | 110 | 71 |
| St Gabriel Fenchurch | 69 | 39 | St Martin Outwich | 60 | 34 |
| St George Botolph-lane | 41 | 27 | St Martin Vintry | 417 | 349 |
| St Gregory by Paul's | 376 | 232 | St Matthew Friday-ftreet | 24 | 6 |
|  |  |  | St Maudlin | | |

|  | Bur. | Pla. |  | Bur. | Pla. |
|---|---|---|---|---|---|
| St Maudlin Milk-ftreet | 44 | 23 | St Olave Hart-ftreet | 237 | 160 |
| St Maudlin Old Fifh-ftreet | 176 | 121 | St Olave Jewry | 54 | 32 |
| St Michael Baffifhaw | 253 | 164 | St Olave Silver-ftreet | 250 | 132 |
| St Michael Cornhill | 104 | 52 | St Pancras Soper-lane | 30 | 15 |
| St Michael Crooked-lane | 179 | 132 | St Peter Cheap | 61 | 35 |
| St Michael Queenhithe | 203 | 122 | St Peter Cornhill | 136 | 76 |
| St Michael Quern | 44 | 18 | St Peter Paul's Wharf | 114 | 86 |
| St Michael Royal | 152 | 116 | St Peter Poor | 79 | 47 |
| St Michael Wood-ftreet | 122 | 62 | St Stephen Coleman-ftreet | 860 | 991 |
| St Mildred Bread-ftreet | 59 | 26 | St Stephen Walbrook | 84 | 17 |
| St Mildred Poultry | 46 | 28 | St Swithin | 93 | 56 |
| St Nicholas Acons | 46 | 28 | St Thomas Apoftle | 163 | 110 |
| St Nicholas Colemby | 125 | 91 | Trinity Parifh | 116 | 79 |
| St Nicholas Olave | 90 | 62 | | | |

Buried in the ninety-feven Parifhes within the Walls — 15207
Whereof of the Plague — 9887

|  | Bur. | Pla. |  | Bur. | Pla. |
|---|---|---|---|---|---|
| St Andrew Holborn | 3958 | 3103 | St George Southwark | 1613 | 1260 |
| St Bartholomew Great | 493 | 344 | St Giles Cripplegate | 8069 | 4838 |
| St Bartholomew Lefs | 193 | 139 | St Olave Southwark | 4793 | 2785 |
| St Bridget | 2111 | 1427 | St Saviour Southwark | 4235 | 3446 |
| Bridewell Precinct | 230 | 179 | St Sepulchre's Parifh | 4509 | 2746 |
| St Botolph Aldergate | 997 | 755 | St Thomas Southwark | 475 | 371 |
| St Botolph Aldgate | 4926 | 4051 | Trinity Minories | 108 | 123 |
| St Botolph Bifhopfgate | 3464 | 2500 | At the Peft-houfe | 159 | 156 |
| St Dunftan Weft | 958 | 665 | | | |

Buried in the fixteen Parifhes without the Walls — 41351
Whereof of the Plague — 28888

|  | Bur. | Pla. |  | Bur. | Pla. |
|---|---|---|---|---|---|
| St Giles in the Fields | 4457 | 3216 | St Magdalen Bermondfey | 1943 | 1362 |
| Hackney Parifh | 232 | 132 | St Mary Newington | 1004 | 1004 |
| St James Clarkenwell | 1803 | 1377 | St Mary Iflington | 696 | 593 |
| St Katherine's Tower | 956 | 601 | St Mary Whitechapel | 4766 | 3855 |
| Lambeth Parifh | 798 | 537 | Rotherhith Parifh | 304 | 210 |
| St Leonard Shoreditch | 2669 | 1949 | Stepney Parifh | 8598 | 6583 |

Buried in the twelve Out-Parifhes in Middlefex and Surrey — 28554
Whereof of the Plague — 21420

|  | Bur. | Pla. |  | Bur. | Pla. |
|---|---|---|---|---|---|
| St Clement Danes | 1969 | 1319 | St Mary Savoy | 303 | 198 |
| St Paul Covent Garden | 408 | 261 | St Margaret Weftminfter | 4710 | 3472 |
| St Martin in the Fields | 4804 | 2883 | Whereof of the Peft-houfe | 156 | 156 |

Buried in the five Parifhes in the City and Liberties of Weftminfter — 12194
Whereof of the Plague — 8403

The Total of all the Chriftenings — 9967
The Total of all the Burials this Year — 97306
Whereof of the Plague — 68596

DISEASE

version of Presbyterianism were not alien. Across the northern Irish province of Ulster a superior quality of life was exemplified by Nova Scotia, and by the western wilderness of North Carolina in the quest for land; indeed, there was the oft-repeated account of the local tacksman. i.e. a Scottish landlord's primary tenant, who acquired vast tracts of land in western Virginia. Across the other three provinces of Ireland, particularly after Cromwell's swift military campaign in 1649, and the re-distribution of property, a chancy trip from Chester and later, from Liverpool, took the risk-taker into a verdant land of sullen, impoverished people. There, land titles were unstable, and fortune favored the bold—especially when the entrepreneur was only lightly impeded by ethics.

In England's southwestern counties, among the people of Wessex whose ancestors had sailed with Drake and Hawkins, looking to the west was not unimaginable; fluctuations in the woolen trade brought them unemployment and worry. The broad, dangerous Atlantic generated trade in several commodities, and ships to transport would-be immigrants sailed from Bristol and other points of departure. While such generalizations about the population which eventually settled the east coastal strip of North America emerge fairly easily, the sense of their lives and the quality of life they perceived individually and internally is harder to gauge.

This essay approaches quality of life stochastically by considering three stages of the process of evolving from emigrants into immigrants, and by inferring attributes generating a sense of the quality of life.

Ideally, one would look to a series of personal diaries, journals, and memoirs; more common are entries in records kept by officers in the ports of departure, and in the records of political units, e.g. county records, which provide documentary evidence of transactions. Bailyn (1985) listed about sixty sources of emigration documents in his multi-phase study of the settling of the east coast of an unexplored continent and the aggregation of British people in North America. Such sources are invaluable, but immigrants bound for Philadelphia, or Baltimore, for example, on their way to settling in prosperous Pennsylvania rarely kept a journal. Life presented more pressing matters day by day.

Once established in the thirteen colonies the proverbial tacksman who acquired a vast acreage needed a way to turn his potential wealth into pounds, shillings and pence. In the years before steam power was available, only the strength of male and female backs, and of animals, was available. To that end a land-rich entrepreneur would order his agents in Britain to recruit young males; women were not necessary at that stage. To cope with the reality that young males would seek the companionship of females; the seventeenth century physician, polymath, and entrepreneur, Sir William Petty (1623–687) proposed that men on his North American properties would be allowed to enter into what he termed "California marriages"—liaisons with native women (Jordan, 2007). That scheme did not mature because Petty lost his lands in 1776.

*Gender.* In time, women with skills were actively recruited as housemaids, milk-maids, and others with useful skills. In addition, there were females who financed their passage in the general hope of bettering the quality of their lives. For some women there was the outcome of marriage and a family, although under circumstances far from what they had been used to. At the time, marriage stressed the practical aspects of a potential union.

*Indenture*. A mechanism by which a poor man or woman might emigrate was the legal contract—the indenture. Nominally a binding agreement, an indenture bound a person to work for a period of years for someone. An indenture drawn up and signed in the county of Middlesex (i.e. the northern environs of the City of London) in the late 1600s specified provision of "Meat, Drink, Apparel, Lodging, and Washing" (Galenson, 1981). The employer might be anyone with money, for the indenture reduced a person to almost a chattel whose services could be sold or bought at will for a price. The essential difference from slavery was the core concept of work to be performed for a fixed but sometimes negotiable period of years. Slavery differed by buying and selling the body of a human being as a chattel.

## 2.2   Personal Factors

After an initial period of unorganized voyaging, emigration and immigration acquired a degree of commercial organization. Agents were designated, ships were adapted to the process, and the flow of emigrants acquired a mercantile style. Across the British Isles agents were charged with recruiting suitable future employees, and persons with the financial resources to set foot on a foreign shore. Until the schism of 1776 the burgeoning colonies received criminals regularly, men and women condemned by the harsh standards of the times to be set down beyond the seas for a specified time. More conventionally, people from various localities recruited under a variety of understandings were aggregated into groups to sail on specified vessels from regionally accessible ports; departure dates were designated irregularly as wind and weather dictated. Equally unpredictable were the routes to the westerly winds of the Atlantic. From Newcastle, for example, Geordies might sail south into the English Channel picking up more voyagers, or north round the top of Scotland and through the maze of Orkney and Shetland islands before facing the broad, rolling waves from the northwest.

Between the agents on both sides of the Atlantic was the ship's captain; he might be an owner engaged in commerce or an opportunist fleecing the unwary migrants. In either case, the ship's captain was the middle agent between the shores of departure and arrival. In all instances money flowed, and human skills and degrees of honesty underwrote what became a commercial enterprise until the fatal, final months before emigration ended in the irreconcilable tensions of 1776 (Table 2.2).

In 1774, the ship *Planter* sailed on the ebb tide on February 2; Captain Daniel Bowers boarded seventy eight indentured men whose destination was Virginia. They ranged in age from twelve to forty seven, with an average I calculate at 26.58 years. The youngest was Joseph Cooley who travelled in a family group headed by his father, Peter, a weaver by trade. There were two other Cooley boys, Peter Jr., age eighteen years, and John age sixteen years. Indentured men usually travelled alone,

**Table 2.2** A model of immigrants' estimated quality of life

| Personal factors | The voyage | The colony |
|---|---|---|
| Gender | Weather | Kith and Kin |
| Age 15–35 | Nearby port | Property |
| Skills | Food at hand | Urban settlement |
| Single | Barber-surgeon | Indenture outcomes |
| Convicted | Sturdy vessel | – *Discharged* |
| Assets | | – *Fled* |
| English-speaking | | – *Cheated* |
| Health | | |
| Gender | | |
| Indenture | | |

although groups who paid for their passage also made the crossing. The Cooleys gave London as their former residence, but that does not mean that they were Londoners. That city may have been the place where they staged, briefly or longer, on the way to Virginia. Many travelers from provincial towns and villages used a two-stage process to North America. It may be noted that some persons walked to London and found work there, or simply returned home discouraged, or recalling the family and connections they had proposed to leave behind. Quality of life, for them, was not fulfilled by the prospects they had foreseen recently in their birthplaces.

In consideration of London "The capital of America" (Flavell, 2010), in the matter of a station on the path to the New World and its hoped-for opportunities, the city was a paradox. Like other urban areas the town had its local versions of viruses for which out-landers had little resistance. London endured a high rate of mortality so that its quality of life was always threatened by the diseases of dirt and poor hygiene. Despite a high rate of mortality the population rebounded as migrants, both permanent and temporary, filled the hiatus in population quickly. The newcomers brought extra-London viruses into the pool of Londoners ("...*born and bred within the sound of Bow bells*"). At all times walking the streets raised the risk of pulmonary tuberculosis spread by coughing, spitting, and sneezing. Those streets and their over-hanging properties maintained their monetary value. From time to time, the metropolitan area was swept by diseases from the Continent. In the years 1593, 1603, 1625, and 1665 plague struck extensively; although the absolute number of deaths was highest in 1665, the rate of mortality as a proportion of all deaths—85.49%—was in 1603 (Jordan, 2017).

Returning to the group of men travelling by indenture, the oldest shipmate for the Cooleys was another weaver, William Siberry, age forty seven years, formerly of London, according to the set of archives for the Port of London identified but not analyzed by Riley (1963). Close to Siberry in age were John Connery, a wig-maker from Southwark who was forty years old. Men like Connery sometimes offered services as a barber/surgeon on the side. Even with John Connery, the *Planter* could provide few medical services to the travelers. This series of indentured men began their travels in a variety of places Some listed a general region, such as a county. Others were more exact naming Durham and Newcastle in the northeast, and sharing a common identity as Geordies. Two men listed in Captain Bowers' records, John Burton, a twenty two year old bricklayer, and Thomas Rand, a butcher of the same age gave un-named places in Ireland as home.

The ship's complement as a whole would have been lucky to travel with John Connery for the weeks of crossing the Atlantic. The Admiralty official, Samuel Pepys, recorded in his first diary that his wigmaker in Westminster failed to check his wig for the fleas found by his wife, Elizabeth. Another indentured man well above the typical indentured servant in age was forty-year old John Harrower. He reached the Port of London from Lerwick in the distant Shetland Islands north of the Scottish mainland. Harrower like the rest, was bound to serve four years; he gave his occupation as clerk and bookkeeper. For the plight of Harower's dependents see the Appendix. Another man well above the typical in age was Peter Collins, a cordwainer.

In the list of declared occupations it was not unknown for indentured men to over-state their skills. Perhaps Edward Fitzpatrick was the surgeon he declared himself to be, or not. It is possible that he was a barber/surgeon choosing to emphasize his valuable if informal skills. It may be noted, in passing, that the port records tersely recorded the presence on board the *Planter* of seventy five other men for whom no details exist. Possibly, they were convicts intended for hard, gang, labor in the colonies, but that observation is merely speculation.

In 1776 the officers of customs and excise closed their registration books in a hiatus which lasted until peace was restored by the events at Yorktown. Slowly, the new peace restored the migration and flow of people on a growing scale exemplified by the influx of German-speaking immigrants from several countries. In theory, the end of an indenture term might lead to compensation in the form of a grant of land, or nothing if the employer were dishonest, as was sometimes the case. A master or a company, for example the Virginia Company, might assemble a group of men and women to work as servants or field workers. An unscrupulous agent might sell his indentured people on the dock when the shipload reached a colonial port. Also, he might march those not sold to the next market town and invite bids for one or more. The work they would perform would depend on the wishes of the new owner and might be far from the work the indentured man or woman anticipated. The word slave is suitable since a bad indenture reduced the person to a veritable slave with few legal rights, except as particular cases were decided in a local court. There were exceptions when a person agreed to an indenture based on specific skills needed in the colonies. Such a person might negotiate a brief period of service, and require particular benefits at the end of the period of service. In such instances the worker specified the terms of service which were enforceable in law. In the case of juveniles, evolving laws protected them, but the vital element in all instances was the relationship to the owner of the indenture.

Not surprisingly, the oppressed worker might abscond and disappear into the general population. Access to shipping might remove a runaway to a different place and so facilitate anonymity. On the other hand, working in a remote site on the western frontier, a servant might have no frame of geographical reference with little or no sense of where he or she was. To flee an oppressive master in the wilderness might be wholly impractical. Balance requires that we acknowledge the instances of indentured men who completed their legal obligations and went on to live successful lives in the colonies. A former period as an indentured servant was not a barrier in a region where many people had settled through that mechanism.

*Age 15–35.* With experience founded in unprofitable investments a colonial agent might reduce his overhead in human beings by providing detailed instructions to his recruiting agent. He would have been conscious of the high mortality which prevailed in the early modem era when epidemics decimated populations. London, a major population center and source of immigrants, was swept by plague in 1665, for example.

One symptom-free young man harboring a communicable disease such as small-pox boarding a ship might infect passengers and crew in the next several weeks, with fatal outcomes in the worst instances. At the best of times, mortality was high in Britain, and higher in the colonies.

Another source of information about conditions in the New World encountered by indentured servants is the set of letters written by young Richard Frethorne born in the parish of St. Dunstan, near the Tower of London into a poor but literate family. The church wardens who exercised secular as well as spiritual functions drew on the processes of the 1601 Poor Law to indenture the young and ship them to the American colonies. This practice saved parish funds, while also implying a brighter future for the youth of the parish. An example from the year 1691 is the following text:

The sonne of William Galloway shalbe put an apprentice unto one

Jeffrey Wallet citizen and carpenter of London now bound for Virginia …

Young Richard Frethorne stepped ashore in Virgina from the ship Abigail at Christmas, 1622. He went to a district called Martin's Hundred, carrying with him the viruses he had acquired on board the Abigail and introducing sickness into the local population, probably including plague which broke out in England with regularity. The year 1603 saw a plague epidemic which generally proved fatal to its victims.

Conditions at Martin's Hundred turned out to be disastrous; one year later, Richard Frethorne wrote a series of letters to his family in St. Dunstan's. From them we can gauge the dreadful conditions he encountered. The purpose of his letters was to use elements of the Poor Law and his relatives' intercessions to finance his release from his indenture. Frethorne wrote:

beseech you and most humble entreat and entirely at your merciful hands …

I am in miserable and pitiful case both for want of meat and want of clothes …

I want clothes for truly I have but one shirt one ragged one, one payer of shoes.

… but one cap …

> Since I came out of the ship I never at anie thing but pease and loblollie (i.e. water gruel).
>
> 4s for deare or venison I never saw anie ... there is some foule but wee are not
>
> Allowed to goe and get yt.
>
> My Cloke is stolen by one of my owne fellowes.. some of my fellowes saw him
>
> Have butter and beife out of a ship, which my Cloke I doubt (not) paid for
>
> What will it bee when wee shall goe a month or two and never see a bit of bread ...
>
> Wee should be turned up to the land and eat barkes of trees or mouldes of the ground.

Concerning the condition of other people working under indentures Frethorne wrote:

> people out day and night, oh that they were in England without their lymbes
>
> and would not care to loose anie lymbe to be in England again.

Recognizing that his relatives needed money to pursue his release from the indenture which had sent him to Virginia Frethome proposed a way to fund his release:

> (if) itt would please yow to send over some beif & some cheese and butter,
>
> or any eating victualles... (there would) be good trading... (!).beg the profits
>
> to redeeeme me.

It seems unlikely that anything came from Frethome's letters. His parents died before his ship reached Virginia (Dahlberg, 2012).

Elsewhere (Jordan, 2012) I have addressed child mortality, a phenomenon in which infants and little children died at a high rate approaching one half in the first five years of life (see Table 1.3). For the survivors, the next cull was the reality of smallpox, a disease which left survivors marked for life by disabilities and skin lesions.

Figure 1.2 shows the generic form of mortality in the early modem era across the life span, a range exceeded today by many people. It indicates how few people were alive at age fifty years (only 346 in a birth cohort of 1348 newborns). Above age fifty years survivors were not the vigorous middle-agers of today, but enfeebled elders probably in poor health and quite dependent on a small donation from the local parish funds. The archives of the parishes of St. Margaret Lothbury in London (Freshfield, 1887), and St. Catherine in Dublin (Jordan, 2017), record charitable acts to the poor. The mechanism was an action by the Vestry, an elected body which acted under the leadership of the parish clergyman; his role expressed his version of charity and the corporal works of mercy, which varied from minister to minister as the spiritual temper of the times changed. The drinking song, "The Vicar of Bray," proclaimed that, "Whatsoever King may reign, still I'll be the Vicar of Bray, Sir." Acts of parish charity ranged from burying a child found dead under a cart, to placing an orphan in foster care with a stipend to the care giver. Typically, the Vestry required that the child be presented to them, quarterly, in good health. Occasionally, a vestry contributed to the cost of passage to the colonies for someone they wished to be gone, a person they considered a public nuisance.

The colonial agent with an eye to his balance sheet requested males between fifteen and thirty five years eliminating males of limited strength and endurance and those past their prime. To indenture a man too weak to clear forest lands in order to create a critical first crop of food on the frontier was impractical. On the other hand, an upper age of thirty five years merely reflected the reality of survival as the seventeenth century evolved into the eighteenth. Tuberculosis and cholera gnawed at the base numbers of the cohort in Fig. 2.3. The number of people alive at age twenty years was 598, and declined to 445 at age forty years, a loss of 153 persons.

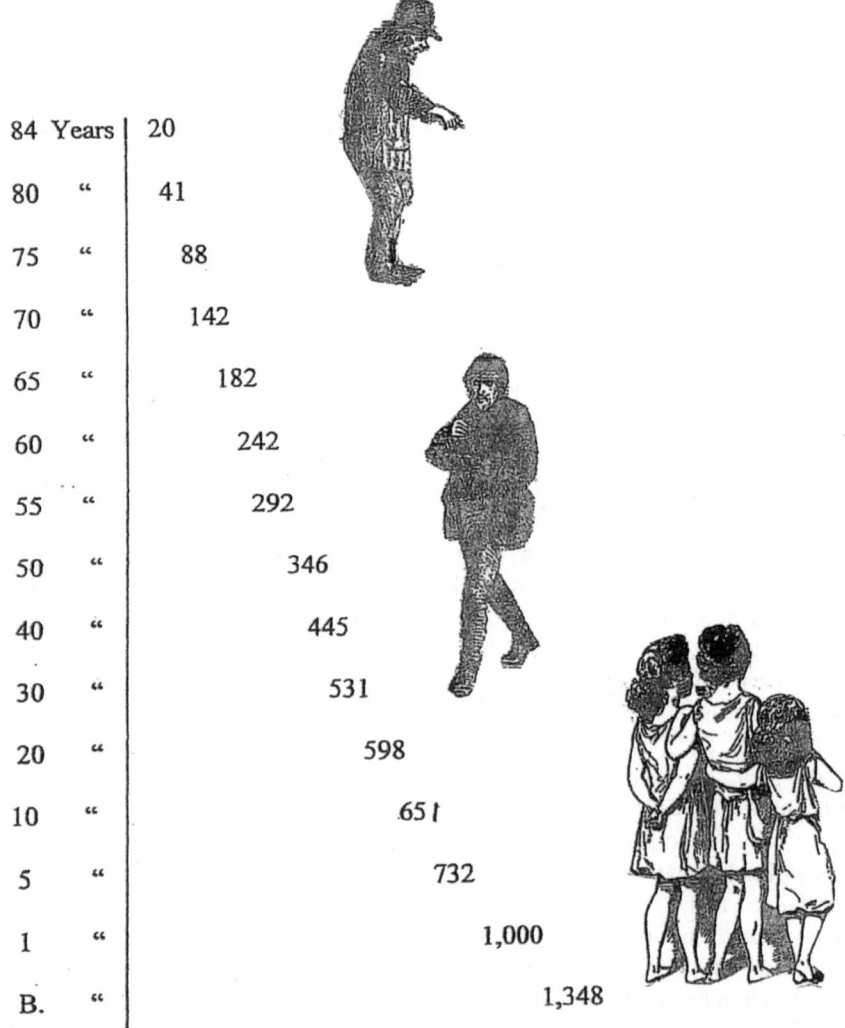

| 84 Years | 20 |
| 80 " | 41 |
| 75 " | 88 |
| 70 " | 142 |
| 65 " | 182 |
| 60 " | 242 |
| 55 " | 292 |
| 50 " | 346 |
| 40 " | 445 |
| 30 " | 531 |
| 20 " | 598 |
| 10 " | 651 |
| 5 " | 732 |
| 1 " | 1,000 |
| B. " | 1,348 |

**Fig. 2.3** Survivorship: birth to age 84 years

Were no age range specified, and considering the same base at age twenty years (N = 598), the number of potential immigrants alive above age fifty declined swiftly. (The numbers are taken from the seventeenth century, but social conditions scarcely moved until well into the nineteenth century.)

One way to understand the slaughter of the elderly would be to say that, with some exceptions, few people entered maturity with the comfort of live grandparents. Colonial agents ensured the quality of life of their work force by excluding would-be immigrants approaching the end of their working lives, a stage which nature culled radically.

*Skills.* In the earliest years of settling the New World it seems that cohorts of immigrants sometimes included too many gentlemen of style, when the reality called for men with practical skills; their talents were used to clear virgin forests, drain swamps, and fend off incursions by autochthonous peoples. Little by little, clearings gave rise to settlements, and then to villages and towns as trading generated a local economy. While for many, especially those with indentures coming to an end, a slow climb up the socio-economic ladder could begin, there were people such as a farmer in Yorkshire's North Riding who liquidated land, cattle, and buildings, and entered the Chesapeake region with cash and a sense of how business was conducted. For such a man, his only disability was his native dialect, one among several regional patterns of speaking which would be difficult to decipher for the many immigrants from London and the adjacent home counties. In the case of German immigrants heading for Pennsylvania, usually in family groups, the use of spoken German, and access to the *Wochentliche Pennsylvanische Staatsbote,* which circulated widely (Bailyn, 1985) were anticipated.

*Single.* In the earliest years strong, vigorous men in their twenties were required as the colonies wrested civilization from the western hills and forests, and the inlets and bays of rivers. Marched in chains, and under guards, men with their vigor as their only asset, were white slaves. In that subculture women were economically inefficient; recruiting agents were instructed to exclude females and to acquire only strong and healthy males in their prime Even their numbers would be decimated by local viruses and accidents.

It is a discrete element, but with the implication of married status as a reciprocal. As the colonies evolved there emerged a place in the social system for housemaids, and women with skills, *e.g.* a milkmaid or a seamstress. Orders came from the New World, over time, for lasses to fill gaps in the structure of families. For example, a widower would never need someone to care for a brood of children. Such a caretaker might be a young relative back in Scotland to whom the colonies offered an improvement in quality of life, and the quality of life of the children would also improve under the care of a relative. Of Course, a woman finding conditions in the colony oppressive might plan to flee her situation in order to escape abuse in several forms.

*Convicted.* An outcome of the events of 1776, was an end to the utility of the colonies as a place to put convicts. Given the harshness of the era's penal code men, women, and children found themselves shipped beyond the seas and condemned to long sentences. The legality within the sentences kept them, like a malevolent virus, at a distance from British society. What their fate was beyond the explicit banishment for many years was beyond the purview of the law at that time. An implication of the system was that transportation was cheaper than building and operating prisons in the United Kingdom. Not until the nineteenth century would Australia and Tasmania become valued sites for dumping criminals of the usual sort involving property and persons. Australia became the relatively genteel exile for the Irish insurgent leader, William Smith O'Brien (Touhill, 1981).

Convict labor could be sold at dockside in Charleston, Philadelphia, Boston, and other colonial sites. Travelling in chains, and probably confined below decks, they arrived in less than optimum health. Dockside sales were held on the deck of the transports, and their services were critical in the early decades of the colonial system. Men who had been sentenced to transportation beyond the seas by the harsh judicial system were a source of profit since they could be sold at the dock. However, probably confined throughout their voyage of several weeks, and cheaply-fed, they were ill-suited for a life of hard labor. In particular, they could be employed as gang labor, and they cleared forests and worked rice paddies until age and ill-health rendered their economic value profitable no longer.

The introduction of African labor eventually became a more efficient investment of capital which reached greater economic and fiscal efficiency when African women conceived, and a generation of children was born into slavery. That aspect amounted to a process of breeding humans, and their acculturation into the life of slavery went more smoothly with their roles in the economy specified by their owners. Convicts, on the other hand, lived with theoretical prospect of an eventual discharge from their labors.

It should be noted that African slaves began to be a better investment for those able to take a long view of the economics of plantation life, including the birth of children into slavery. The arrival of convict labor declined as slavery took its place. Immigration from the British Isles grew across the eighteenth century, and so did the importation of unwilling immigrants; a canny ship-owner arranged transportation of legal slaves in groups, whether male or female, to the West Indies and continental colonies to the north. The instrumental concept, quality of life, scarcely applies to people bought and sold like so many beasts of burden. Even their plight saw an improvement when religion entered their lives, and with it the infusion of literacy. The latter became a key to entering the world of literature and its revolutionary concepts of freedom and other liberating—if tantalizing -scenarios.

*Assets*. Unlike the stereotype of an immigrant as a person without assets and desperately poor There were people who had wealth. In Ireland, "the Ulster custom" permitted liquidation of improvements. A tenant farmer could liquidate his possessions in the form of cattle and equipment. Such a step arose when, for example, a property owner enjoying the delights of fashionable Bath, earnest Edinburgh, or cosmopolitan London, decided to erect a fine country house; he raised his rental income and enclosed what had been common grazing land. When rents became intolerable and the renters fled, evicting landlords lost income; as a class, they sought ineffectively to stop emigration to the colonies.

To the many artisans with skills the regions adjoining Chesapeake Bay and the Hudson river offered opportunities to participate in their growth, and to earn higher wages. In Bailyn's (1985) study, about ninety occupations in six categories were recorded for people in the broad category of indentured servants. On the other hand, a youngest son might have few prospects in the Scottish highlands and be dispatched to the New World by the Laird with a little capital.

*English-speaking*. Initially, the majority of immigrants spoke English, the exceptions being Highland Scots and residents of the western islands, and, later, German-speaking immigrants from the Continent. The common bond among the majority meant that they entered the New World familiar with the major elements of the new society. The majority were English, and as indentured workers, or not, they knew that there was a body of civil and criminal law, and that contracts were enforceable. Dissolving that certainty to a degree was their grasp of the sociology of power in which the privileged often had their way at the expense of their social inferiors. The immigrants were typically English men and women moving into a society of other English men and women; it was, however, a new society in which evolution and change were well under way, and the premises of the old country were changed by facts predominant on the frontier, and a natural order in which disease and weather set the boundaries of daily life. The institutions of the colonies were molded in their evolution by the binding force of the shared language of speech and literature-English. Of course, there were outlayers; for example, it is likely that some of the travelers departing through the inland port of Bristol spoke Welsh, or the Cornish language, a Celtic tongue whose last speaker lived until the early nineteenth century, and there were the natives of the western zones of Scotland who were Gaelic speakers, and in some places Catholic.

*Health*. In other studies (Jordan, 1993b, 2013, 2017), I have explored the risks to life and limb encountered by people. In the early modern era it is likely that many people were sick. Walking down the street in London, Edinburgh, Dublin, and Bristol meant moving amidst clouds of invisible viruses. For those whose immediate objective was moving to the local centers of population exposure to unfamiliar microbes was probable; the result was that the first stage of the emigration process, reaching a port of embarkation, could be a health hazard.

Setting aside the risk of facing non-local viruses there were infections ranging from local variants of common diseases. For children there was the expectation that they would run the gauntlet of smallpox, a disease which might kill a child or leave behind a sequelae of damages to the senses and skin lesions. Not until the nineteenth century would scarlet fever begin to mutate into the important but non-fatal children's disease we know today. At all times and places there lurked the invisible killer tuberculosis. That condition presented symptoms as thoracic and glandular, the latter known as the King's Evil was thought curable by the king's touch, among the superstitious.

A number of life-threatening diseases—typhus, for example—shared the common trait of being rooted in dirt. There were illnesses spread by personal lack of cleanliness in which lack of hygienic practices such a neglect of wigs among gentlemen and hair care among ladies set the stage for vermin-spread diseases. At the community level there was a lack of sanitation and toilet waste was poorly disposed of.

Fear of disease was universal, and some diseases arrived as epidemics. Cholera is an example, and bubonic plague decimated urban populations; that swift killer struck London several times in the early modem era. It broke out in 1593,1603, 1625, and 1665. Given the speed with which the infected died a rough screening by a ship's captain could identify plague victims. However, it is not hard to imagine a case of plague destroying passengers and crew swiftly once a ship left port and reached the broad Atlantic. Cholera was no less a threat to an emigrant group. Amidst the social disorganization of an epidemic, wealth and social status were irrelevant. Rich and poor died from diseases of filth, and from those transmitted by coughing and sneezing. It seems likely that a ship's captain would refuse to accept even a fully paid up emigrating passenger burdened with a serious cough, or appearing to be ill. However, such vigilance would be ineffective when a passenger brought on board the bacillus which we know as tuberculosis (Fig. 2.4).

## 2.3   The Voyage

*Weather*. In the early modem era the passage from western Europe to the New World was well established. For the Portuguese the fishing grounds of the Grand banks were familiar, and the Spaniards established their hegemony to the south quickly. From the British Isles the course took vessels by a route that went south and west towards the Azores and, and then due west as the trade winds dictated. The passage to Nova Scotia encountered the great green waves of the north Atlantic, rather than the more gentle winds off the Azores heading west. Some emigrant ships sailed easily across the broad Atlantic, while others simply vanished. Over time navigation charts pointed out the few landmarks, such as the Scilly Isles west of Land's End where wrecks were frequent. Civilians making the voyage recalled the fate of Sir Cloudsley Shovell in 1707, and the loss of fifteen hundred hands on the rocks and shoals of the Scyillies when returning to England.

Typically, we turn to a practitioner of a trade to gauge its impact on those who practice it, and on the quality of life experienced by those in the trade. In the case of travelling by sea in the early modem period practitioners were men who served before the mast- probably illiterate and far from literary enthusiasms. There are rare exceptions to be noted, but they wrote of splices, masts, and sails. A work of that genre was the journal of John Grimshaw who sailed under Admiral Horatio Nelson in the Mediterranean. His ship was the 74-gun, *HMS Vanguard*, and he began his entries on 24 December, 1797 (see Jordan, 2003).

# LONDONS
## LAMENTATION.
### Or a fit admonifhment for City
### and Countrey,

Wherein is defcribed certaine caufes of this affliction and vi
fitation of the Plague, yeare 1641. which the Lord hath
been pleaf-d to inflict upon us,and withall what meanes
muft be ufed to theLord,to gaine his mercy and favor,
with an excellent fpirituall medicine to be ufed
for the prefervative both of Body and Soule.

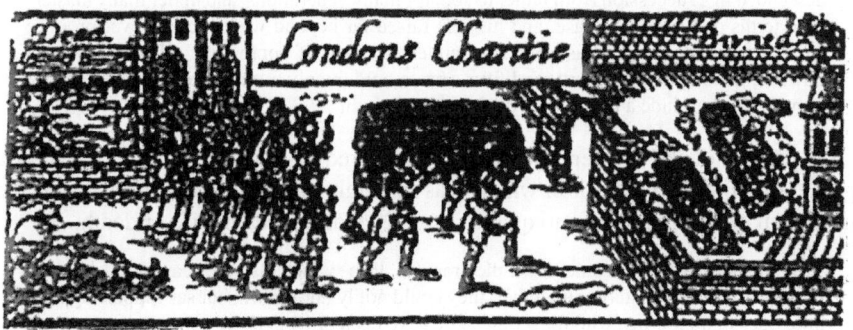

London, Printed by E. P. for Iohn Wright Junior. 1641.

**Fig. 2.4** Burying London's dead

Twenty five years earlier, an Edinburgh lady, Ms. Janet Schaw (Andrews and Andrews, 1921) began a journal on 25 October, 1774 as she began an odyssey of seven weeks across the Atlantic to the West Indies and, eventually, to North Carolina. The occasion for the voyage was to accompany her brother on his way to assume a post as a customs official in the harbor at St. John's, Antigua. Ms. Schaw and her brother, plus a friend's children, were to be the sole passengers but, one day, having sailed around the north of Scotland, they heard voices and witnessed a group of people boarding their ship, the *Jamaica Packet.* The owner, George Parker, had instructed the Captain to smuggle aboard this group of emigrants who had indentured themselves to Parker.

Ms. Schaw gave us a literate and cultured person's impression of the immigrants.

> I saw the deck covered with people of all ages, from three weeks old to three score, men, women, children and suckling infants. Never did my eyes behold so wretched, so disgusting a sight. They looked like Dean Swift's Yahoos newly caught. They were fully as sensible of the motion of the vessel, and sickness works more ways than one, so that, so that the smell which came from the hole, where they had been confined, was sufficient to raise a plague aboard.

Among the wretched immigrants were two people Ms. Schaw came to know, Mr. and Mrs. Lawson, and so addressed by the other immigrants.

> ...till lately, in very affluent circumstances. He rented a considerable farm, which had descended in a succession from father to son, for many generations, and under many masters .The terms of Lawson's Lease. and his rent raised far beyond what it could ever produce .he was forced to give up his all to the unrelenting hand of oppression... I have just seen Lawson, he is a, between forty and fifty...has a bold, manly, weather beaten countenance .turning away to hide a tear, which did him no discredit ...

A portrait of the women and children appeared in Ms. Schaw's journal after a period of more than a week in which seas ran high, and living conditions reached a minimum of quality, in fact no quality at all as quality became life or death.

> ... without air but what came down the crannies, thro' which also the sea poured on them incessantly. For many days altogether, they could not ly (sic) down, but sat supporting their little ones in their arms, who must otherwise have been drowned.

For the Shaw party life was not much better. Ms. Schaw recalled the effects of one storm.

> ... the cabin door burst open and I was overwhelmed with an immense wave, which broke my chair from its moorings, floated everything in the Cabin and I found myself swimming among joint-stools, chests, Tables and all the various furniture of our parlour.here comes the Captain. He says, he expects a hard gale.

The experience of crossing the Atlantic was a great leveler bringing encounters among people of all levels of gentility. Space was designed for cargo rather than people. The man who leased the *Jamaica Packet,* Alexander Schaw, slept in a hammock, and the stateroom (as it was represented to Schaw) was only five feet by six feet, and two people slept there in bunks.

But the *Jamaica Packet* and her band of immigrants prevailed. After reaching the trade winds they sailed smoothly to the West Indies, and then turned north to Wilmington, in the Carolinas. Ms. Schaw sailed east to Lisbon on the *Rebecca* where our contact through her journal ends. Nothing is known of her life other than that she returned to Edinburgh, the Athens of the North, in due course. Of the emigrants from Scotland even less is known.

Ms. Schaw's journal described terrifying scenes, and Nature and Davy Jones were always a threat. On the other hand, commercial considerations improved the process of trans-Atlantic travel. In 1740 a religious leader in Savannah, Georgia, invited one of the leading lights of Methodism, the Reverend George Whitfield, to preach there, beginning a series of trans-Atlantic roundtrips until his death in New England in 1770.

*Nearby Port.* For farmers and others in the North Riding of Yorkshire intending to make the hazardous voyage to the New World their hegira began by getting to a port of embarkation. Such places on the coast of the North Sea were exemplified by Newcastle, Whitby, and Hull.

Walking to the port of embarkation side of Scotland, and close to Glasgow, Burnt Island, on the Firth of Forth to the east was a choice of desperation for them. To the south, would-be immigrants in the counties around the capital city used the Pool of London. In the southwestern counties Bristol was the choice, and emigrants from the hinterlands used the port of London. Getting to Whitby from a village or rural farm in the North Riding of the northern county, Yorkshire, might, for the fortunate, entail renting a coach to travel along rough roads.

For the ordinary young man intending to serve an indenture, a hard walk of several days awaited. To finance his travel, a hypothetical tailor Jan Pierce, sold his remaining asset, his grey mare, to Tom Hardy. For many people emigration began on foot, and there would have been challenges such as meals and safe resting places across Wessex to Bristol (Souden, 1978).

The quality of life when accessing the port of departure depended on the immigrant's age and health, and the children of the poor experienced stress proportional to their age. For all ages, travel to the port of departure meant passage through places they might have heard of, but in an era when life was a local affair new places and sub-populations meant exposure to local hostilities, non-local viral strains and the high rates of crime. Thus the health of ship-board travelers was framed to a degree before they even reached the port of departure, or glimpsed the vessel which would be their home for two to three months at sea, or their graves. The first phase of a multi-part undertaking was no less dangerous than the second. Part of this phase of emigration was being processed by port authorities in procedures which varied by place and time. In some ports the authorities developed records useful in our generation as we reconstruct the flow of emigration and estimate the migrants' quality of life in their hegira, London and Bristol have been productive in this regard; both ports were centers of population in the immediate urban sense, but also as regional centers of commerce serving local and international business interests.

Once the immigrants from the provinces reached London the Captain would leave on ebb tide for the New World; the traveler might succumb to London's attractions joining the permanent floating population, or find work in the urban complex and decide to settle there; internal migration was a fairly common practice in search of work (Clark, 1979). Of course settling in the great port city also meant not returning to Grantham or whichever place had seen the traveler contemplate a better quality of life. Curiosities of the pre-industrial era were the remote spots from which some journeys had begun, e.g. John Harrower from the Shetland Islands.

*Food at hand*. In the mind's eye we see a migrant—let us call him Jan Pierce—making his way from Colyton, in Devonshire, to the port of emigration, Bristol. He brought food to sustain him as he walked a considerable distance towards the place and time of his transatlantic voyage. Use of food from home was an economy vital to his travel. No less critical were the arrangements for his food for the months he would be at sea. Then Shetland indentured clerk John Harrower bought and sold small items to pay for food—typically bread, cheese and beer (Riley, 1963) on his search for a ship.

For a family travelling together deck space was covered with their live chickens, pigs, and other beasts in cages, apart from spars, extra sails, and equipment to maintain the vessel. An alternative was to rely on the ship's owner or captain to provide food. Such reliance on a stranger engaged in commerce of a dubious nature, at best, and having absolute control of supplies and personnel, was a decision those sailing from Burnt Island in the Firth of Forth with Ms. Schaw came to regret. For indentured servants provision of food was a part of the legal relationship, but it was not one always honored fully by the owner or ship's captain.

*Barber-Surgeon*. Should illness strike down a person travelling to the New World the possibility of receiving care was slim; the sole exception was sea-sickness, an affliction which struck one immigrant while Ms. Schaw's ship was still tied to the dock. Until the nineteenth century, the practice of medicine was largely based, like the practice of law, in an apprentice system. In England, the highest level of professional qualification was membership in the Royal College of Physicians, a qualification difficult to attain. The physician and polymath, Dr. William Petty, was recognized while still quite young in broadsheet newspapers and other forms of expression, as the Oxford Professor of Medicine who revived the woman hanged at Oxford for infanticide and abortion, Nan Green. Petty waited almost a decade until death of a Fellow created a vacancy in the College's roll of approved physicians, despite his reputation.

The ordinary man or woman would have sought the services of a barber-surgeon. Such persons, along with pharmacists, herbalists, apothecaries, empirics, and others dealt with broken limbs, teeth extractions, and the many disorders which responded to alcohol-fortified liquids. An example was the widely used tonic introduced in the 1640s and known by his name, the Rev. Thomas Daffy, whose elixir spread when a relative moved to London and introduced Daffy's Elixir to the population. With its high alcohol content this *"Elixir Salutis"* eased many a pain (Fig. 2.5).

The limited pharmacy on a ship probably consisted of alcohol-based remedies. Should a physician or barber-surgeon be sailing to the New World to start a practice in, say, New York or Philadelphia, indentured shipmates would be unusually fortunate. Being a barber-surgeon was a sideline to a business offering other services, in many cases. A wig maker or a pharmacist might set limbs and pull teeth on the side.

A curiosity of the pre-industrial era was the compounding of ointments from smelly, obscure items which resembled Shakespeare's "fillet of a fenny snake." In that regard, obtaining a prescription from a Fellow of the Royal College or a barber-surgeon would have been equally ineffective, but far more expensive. In the case of a physician's prescription, the error would have been compounded by his rationale derived from the doctrine of the humours, or from consulting Nicholas Culpeper's *Pharmacopoeia Londinensis*. The cover of this work notes him as *"Gent."*

*Sturdy Vessel.* The longest immigrant voyage began on a comparatively small merchant ship designed for trade, one smaller than the increasingly large, complicated men o'war exemplified by H.M.S. *Hercules.* The Hollanders' refined their merchant fleet into efficient vessels sailing east to the trading zone known as the Dutch East Indies and controlled, in Holland's golden age, by the East India Company.

To understand the state of shipping in the United Kingdom (as the nation would be known after the Act of Union with Scotland in 1707) it is helpful to consider the people's state of mind, their perception of the physical world, what Maruyama (1980) termed their *mindscapes*. In the pre- industrial years curiosity was not a virtue, and conservatism prevailed in all fields. Only slowly did empiricism bring the microscope, and the images generated by Robert Hooke gain acceptance. As early as the years of James I and VI, a submarine had been demonstrated in the Thames, and a steam engines of sorts presented.

In those two and similar instances, the innovations were seen as amusing, but little more. When William Petty demonstrated his double-bottom boat—a catamaran, Samuel Pepys and Lord William Brouncker, President of the Royal Society and friend of the Stuart brothers, were about the only people of influence who were impressed. Petty built several versions of his double-bottom before his death in 1687. In the eighteenth century ship design began to evolve, extending keels, simplifying rigging and sails, and reducing crews; these innovations improved the economics of building and operating ships, but wind and weather undermined rational innovation in designing ships, *vide* Petty's "double-bottom" vessel which was fast and highly steerable.

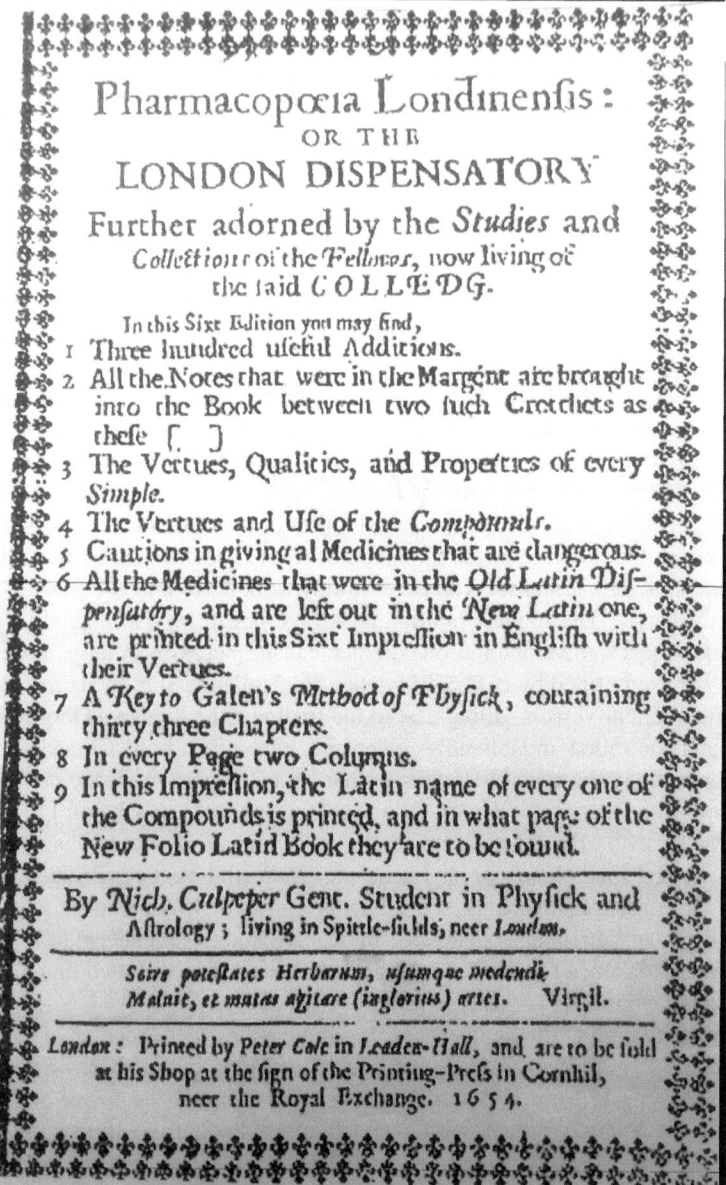

**Fig. 2.5** *Pharmacopoeia Londinensis*

## 2.4 The Colonies

*Kith and Kin.* Eventually, the immigrants reached a port on the east coast of North America. There, a hypothetical Jan Pierce, an indentured tailor with some skills as a cobbler, met his future. Along with his fellow travelers he found himself bewildered by the bustle along the quay, its noises, and the complexity he glimpsed in the town spreading along the riverside; also he encountered the heat of a Spring day in the New World and the profusion of plant life along the river banks. An immigrant, if fortunate, might connect here with kith and kin in a pattern of chain migration. Such re-connection boded well for the prospects of newcomers.

With his indenture specifying vaguely his experience and skill and lined up on the deck with other men, the tailor found himself inspected by would-be purchasers of his contract—"soul drivers," to work for three years. With his indenture purchased by a fellow tailor his work for the immediate future was settled. For some immigrants the fare to cross the ocean was paid by use of a down-payment; the *redemptioner,* a skilled worker for example, would freelance for a few weeks and pay off the balance, or perhaps his indenture. In the case of our hypothetical tailor from Colyton, in Devon, he had in mind that he might work off his contract in the Chesapeake Bay region, of which people in the county of Devon had heard good things, but he learned a little before landing that the ship was near Wilmington, in the Carolinas. Determination of latitude necessary to place a vessel accurately on a chart was slow to spread, dependent on the use of an accurate and expensive time-piece

Where a number of Scots had settled and prospered, he took in several items. There were black African slaves working on the docks. people he had not seen before. He wondered if their blackness would rub off onto him if he worked with them. Also, despite the belief held in Colyton that America was populated with dark-skinned people, he found that the locals were white and spoke English. In time, the immigrant was helped in his integration by familiarity with the conventions of his homeland, now institutionalized in the maturing colonies and nominally governed by a London-appointed Governor. The employment experience was beyond the control of the indentured men, most of whom were servants of one kind or another. The Wilmington agents inspected newly arrived men in order to fill requests for particular skills. The system matured over the years so that, with time, brute force as an arrival's asset changed, and the maturing colony needed technical skills such as fabricating jewelry, being a chef rather than a cook. and skill at joinery such as inlay work in mahogany. Female skills such as child care, needle work, and hairdressing were sought in the later years.

What we may loosely call character entered into the situation of immigrants who were unencumbered. Within their natures were traits—some acquired, some innate—in the form of needs or drives. For example, within some landed immigrants there was a strong drive to succeed which showed itself in achievement of several sorts. It existed in the form of a sense of excellence which, one hopes, had not been extinguished by indenture, or by the hardships of the voyage, or Table 2.3 provides a numerical glance at the selective way immigrants viewed their future location;

**Table 2.3** Destinations of indentured servants, in rank order, 1654–1775 (N = 11,773)

| | Virginia | Maryland | Pennsylvania | Carolina | New England | New-York | New Jersey |
|---|---|---|---|---|---|---|---|
| Males | 5461 | 3322 | 955 | 85 | 38 | 38 | |
| M/F ratio | 3.4:1 | 8.3:1 | 9.5:1 | 8.5:1 | 3.2:1 | 9.5:1 | |
| Females | 1650 | 462 | 105 | 10 | 33 | 4 | |
| Percentage | 60 | 29 | 9 | <0.01 | <0.01 | <0.01 | |

[a]Developed from Galenson (1981), pp. 221–223

though whether or not the indented workers reached their hoped-for goal was partly due to weather and chance. In the United Kingdom literature on the colonies and reports from visitors circulated. Agents developed materials on the prospects they offered, especially in the area where the agents' American patrons sought servants with particular skills.

Instances of indentures persisted into the twentieth century; There is the verified example of a man living in central Europe, in the 1920s, whose indenture required him to work as a lumberjack in Canada. He accepted the terms of indenture in order to cross the Atlantic and reach North America. In stages, over several years, he made his way and joined the Czech community in a large Midwestern city in the United States.

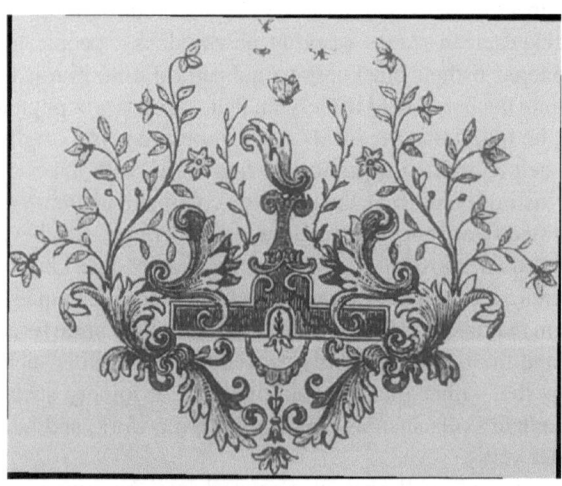

## Appendix 1: John Harrower's Wife and Bairns and the Plight of an Emigrant Male's Dependents

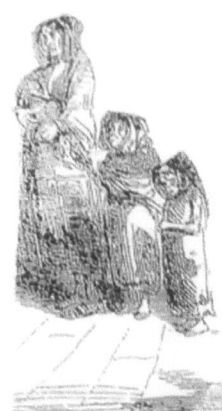

| Age in years | Survivors |
|---|---|
| 20 " | 598 |
| 10 | 651 |
| 5 | 732 |
| 1 | 1,000 |
| Birth | 1,348 |

John Graunt's Life Table

Viz of 100 there dies within the first six years … 36 The next ten years, or Decade … 24 The second Decad … 15. The third Decad…08 The Fourth … 6 the next …3 The next …2 The next …1

From whence it follows, that of the said 100 conceived there remains alive at six years end 64. At Sixteen years end … 40 At 26… 25

At tirty (sic) … 16 At Fourty six …10 At fifty six …6 At sixty six …3 At seventy six…1 At eighty …()

(Graunt, 1662, p. 70)

## Appendix 2: Numerical Estimate of Females Indentured to America, Quality of Life

| Domain | Rating | | | | |
|---|---|---|---|---|---|
| | −2 | −1 | 0 | +1 | +2 |
| Gender (M) | ☹ | | | | |
| Skills | | | | | ☹ |
| Single | | | | | ☺ |
| Convicted | | | | | |

(continued)

(continued)

| Domain | Rating | | | | |
|---|---|---|---|---|---|
| | −2 | −1 | 0 | +1 | +2 |
| Assets | | | | | ☺ |
| English-speaking | | | | | ☺ |
| Prior health | | ☹ | | | |
| Nearby port | | | | ☺ | |
| New climate | | | ? | | ☺ |
| Food at hand | | | | ☺ | |
| Barber-surgeon, physician, herbalist, *et alii* | | | | | ☺ |
| Sturdy vessel | | | | | ☺ |
| Kith and kin | | | | | ☺ |
| Property | | | | | ☺ |
| Urban settlement | | | | | ☺ |

## Appendix 3: Numerical Estimate of Males Indentured to America, Quality of Life

| Domain | Rating | | | | |
|---|---|---|---|---|---|
| | −2 | −1 | 0 | +1 | +2 |
| Gender (M) | | | | | ☺ |
| Skills | | | ○ | | |
| Single | | | | ☺ | |
| Convicted | | ☹ | | | |
| Assets | | | | | ☺ |
| English-speaking | | | | ☺ | |
| Health | | | ○ | | |
| Weather | | | ○ | | |
| Nearby port | | | | ☺ | |
| Food at hand | | | | | ☺ |
| Barber/surgeon | | | | | ☺ |
| Sturdy vessel | | | | | ☺ |
| Kith and kin | | | | | ☺ |
| Property | | | ○ | | |
| Urban settlement | | | | | ☺ |

(continued)

(continued)

| Domain | Rating | | | | |
|---|---|---|---|---|---|
| | −2 | −1 | 0 | +1 | +2 |
| *Indenture* | | | | | |
| – Discharged | | | | | |
| – Fled | | | | ☺ | |
| – Cheated | | | | ☹ | |

# References

Andrews, E. W., Andrews, C. M. (1921). *Journal of a lady of quality*. New Haven, CT: Yale University Press.

Bailyn, B. (1985). *Voyagers to the West*. New York: Knopf.

Clark, P. (1979). Migration in England during the late seventeenth and early eighteenth centuries. *Past and Present, 83*, 81–90.

Dahlberg, S. L. (2012). "Do not forget me": Richard Frethorne, indentured servitude, and the English Poor Law of 1601. *Early American Literature, 47*, 1–30.

Flavell, J. (2010). *When London was capital of America*. New Haven, CT: Yale University Press.

Freshfield, E. (1887). *The Parish registries of St. Margaret Lothbury*. London: Parish Register Society.

Galenson, D. W. (1981). *White servitude in colonial America: An economic analysis*. Cambridge: Cambridge University Press.

Graunt, J. (1662). *Natural and political observations mentioned in a following index, and made upon the bills of mortality*. London: Martin, Allestry, and Dicas.

Jordan, T. E. (1993a). *The degeneracy crisis and Victorian youth*. Albany, NY: SUNY Press.

Jordan, T. E. (1993b). Stay and starve or go and prosper! Juvenile emigration from Great Britain in the nineteenth century. *Social Science History, 9*, 145–166.

Jordan, T. E. (2003). *With Nelson at the Nile*. Naval History 32–33.

Jordan, T. E. (2007). *A copper farthing: Sir William Petty (1623–1687) and his times*. Sunderland (UK): University of Sunderland Press.

Jordan, T. E. (2012). *Quality of life and mortality among children: historical perspectives*. New York: Springer.

Jordan, T. E. (2013). Victorian Britain and the quality of life. In A. C. Michalos (Ed.), *Encyclopedia of quality of life research*. New York: Springer.

Jordan, T. E. (2017). *Quality of life and mortality in seventeenth century London and Dublin*. New York: Springer.

Maruyama, M. (1980). Mindscapes and science theories. *Current Anthropology, 21*, 589–599.

Riley, E. W. (1963). *The journal of John Harrower: An indentured servant in the colony of virginia: 1773–1776*. New York: Holt, Rinehart, and Winston.

Souden, D. (1978). Rogues, whores, and Vagabonds? indentures servant immigrants...of mid-seventeenth Bristol. *Social History, 3*, 23–29.

Touhill, B. M. (1981). *William Smith O'Brien and his Revolutionary Companions in Exile*. Columbia, MO: University of Missouri Press.

# Chapter 3
# Forced Emigration to the Antipodes

**Abstract** This Chapter examines the quality of life experienced by men, women, and boys who, unlike the migrants bound for America, moved eastward in a long, frequently solitary voyage. These emigrants did not move voluntarily, within a growing stream of more conventional migrants, for they were male, female, and boy felons. With rare exceptions their origins were from the ranks of the urban poor, and tended not to be first-time offenders. Several transport ships of the early Victorian era are considered.

**Keywords** Australia · First fleet · *Emma Eugenia* · Point Puer · Hobart · William Smith O'brien

## 3.1 Preface

The age of sail ended, like most social processes, as a transition from one age to another. It did so at a time of vigorous innovation in technology when British society was static, and natural disasters and upheavals in distant places were reported from "abroad."

In the case of the age of sail, the British Isles were well supplied with wooden ships and sails which yielded nostalgia to emerging technology. The Royal navy was large and exerted influence in many parts of the world. A wooden ship of the line was expensive to build in processes hallowed by tradition. As the nineteenth century opened, for example, Admiral Horatio's flagship, H.M.S. *Victory*, was already more than a half-century old, and she serves today—although laid up in dry dock at Portsmouth.

Inevitably, the emerging practicality of steam and screw in the service of commerce infiltrated commercial shipping. Early applications were in wooden boats with paddles. That stage was followed by construction using metal sheets to form steel hulls. By 1838, a date in an era to be considered to be considered shortly, the wooden ship *Sirius*, powered by steam crossed the Atlantic comparatively indifferent to the direction of the wind. Shortly after, the steamship, *Great Western*, using screw propellers rather than paddles, crossed the Atlantic.

© The Author(s), under exclusive license to Springer Nature Switzerland AG 2020        47
T. Jordan, *Quality of Life and Early British Migration*,
SpringerBriefs in Well-Being and Quality of Life Research,
https://doi.org/10.1007/978-3-030-33077-4_3

By the time the cohort of men, women, and boys examined in this chapter matured the maritime affairs of the British Isles epitomized to the Victorians the possibilities of steam and steel, although wind, currents, and sails prevailed until fuel supplies around the globe were assured to supply the "Moloch of Steam."

All of this growth and change was not without its social price, and I treated that topic in, The Degeneracy Crisis and Victorian Youth (1993b). Across the Irish Sea Ireland under Queen Victoria's governments proved resistant to Westminster's designs, but it was a fruitful place to recruit Ireland's young men for the thin red line in far-off places. The most geographically remote places on the planet, apart from the poles, were the Antipodes—Australia, Tasmania, and New Zealand.

The people crossing the Atlantic and those about to be discussed,—people dispatched by the law to the south Pacific—had several things in common. Criminality, as defined by law at the time was a shared element for people crossing the Atlantic, and making the lengthy voyage, to Australia. For both sets of emigrants, the ocean, travel, and life on a sailing ship, were shared elements.

## 3.2   Victorian Britain

Table 1.5 provided a summary of conditions in the nineteen century; however, that quantitative portrait may be expanded by getting closer to the lives of Victorian people in the early and middles decades of an age of sail but also one of innovations in technology.

The early years of the nineteenth century were dominated by the Napoleonic Wars which ended with the defeat of the French at Waterloo in 1815. The political consequences were good and national security was assured. On the other hand, peace ended the need for material supports for the war effort, and widespread economic distress followed. One outcome of peace was the emergence of a "super abundant agricultural pauper population for whose labour no adequate demands exist," in the language of a Parliamentary committee (Carrier & Jeffery, 1953). While rural life deteriorated, urban dwellers also struggled as the Corn Laws protecting farmers' interests kept high the price people paid for bread; that situation prevailed until Prime Minister Robert Peel ended the corn laws in 1846.

The situation of urban dwellers was tied to the rise of factories. Application of steam power, at once visible energy and noisy, made the rise of manufactures a symbol of the entire century. Residents of Birmingham, Manchester, and Leeds toiled amidst harsh conditions.

The propertied class found that income from the agricultural products of the soil were matched by profits from under the same soil. The country's geology consisted in many places, of coal. That mineral was excavated in mines whose extraction was the product of labor at the coal face, a locus of total darkness, accumulation of dangerous gases, and the risk of structural collapse. In that satanic setting labored men, women, and children. With only small miner's lamps to illuminate the coal face and little or no ventilation coal was extracted under appalling conditions. Ordinary folk tried to organize into bargaining units, but unions were illegal, as the fate of the Tolpuddle martyrs made clear. Small towns arose around the extraction of coal in many places. A series of reports from factory Commissioners built a picture of poverty and deprivation which shattered the consciences of thoughtful people (Fig. 3.1).

In factories conditions were different, but no less harmful; long hours, unprotected machinery, and harsh discipline were the themes of factory life. The quality of life for all but the middle and upper classes was poor. The consciences of some observers were outraged, and the years saw the emergence of a set of observers and reformers. In Manchester conditions of life and work in the manufacture of cotton goods were set forth by Karl Marx and his disciple, Friedrich Engels. There were reformers who sought remediation of social evils. Also committed to reform and to philanthropy for Lancashire mill workers was James Kay-Shuttleworth.

In the nineteenth century there emerged the reformers, Edward Brenton, Mary Carpenter, Lord Shaftesbury (Anthony Ashley Cooper), Leonard Horner, William Booth, and Thomas Barnardo, among others. That is not to say that reformers were always successful, and scandal-free; some of the child-saving organizations could

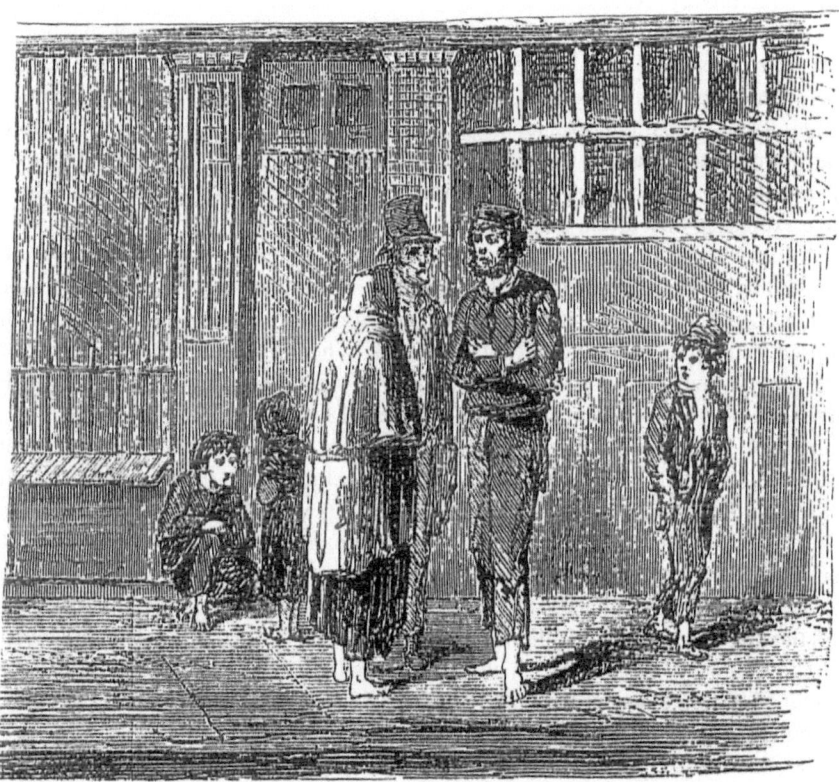

**Fig. 3.1** A mid-Victorian street scene

be high-handed, and efforts to rescue alcoholics from their plight often failed in individual circumstances.

Occasionally, there were liberal-minded factory owners. Robert Owen, of New Lanark had a utopian streak in his management philosophy and he introduced reforms on the factory floor. To work for Owen was to engage in physical exercise, and to attend lectures while on the payroll. Later in the century, factory owners built housing for workers, a venture which provided social control of working people while also generating substantial returns on the investment; an example is Titus Salt who constructed Saltaire, near Leeds. Charles Dickens contributed to the philanthropic literature with the Cheeryble brothers based on the Grant brothers in Lancashire. Balance requires mention of Alexander Ure whose 1835 book, The Philosophy of Manufactures, reasoned that the factory floor was an indulgent site.

In the 1840s Nature devastated Ireland when the summer crop of the potato developed a fungus which killed the plant, and which spread rapidly. Throughout that episode, Ireland exported food, and the poor who lived outside the economy did not have cash to purchase foodstuffs.

There followed harsh decisions leading to large scale emigration, largely to British cities and to North America.

Across the British Isles, tea became a popular beverage at a time when alcoholism was a serious social issue. In Table 3.1 about one quarter of the three family budgets was spent on bread and potatoes. Inquiry is guided by the values of any generation. It is unfortunate but understandable that the study of those household expenditures was not repeated at a later date; such inquiry repeated once or several times, would have yielded a temporal-sequential account of expenditure; such information would have expressed the current quality of domestic life.

A challenge to the consumer-housewife across the Victorian era was the hazard of adulterated food. The risk to peoples' health was considerable as overly aggressive entrepreneurs sought to extract the last farthing from the foods and sundries the offered to the public. That domestic challenge to health sometimes ended in death. The poor sometimes enrolled newborns in one or more insurance schemes; at the time, death was a frequent visitor to families. Table 3.2 views death of the most vulnerable in numerical terms; across the fifteen years 1841–1855, mortality events were largely stable, recalling that the period includes the "Hungry Forties." The mortality rate for those under one year was high, by twenty first century expectations. Little systematic recording of mortality rates was extant, although the reality of death fell as age increased. Chadwick's sanitary initiatives undoubtedly saved lives over the years. On the other hand, clinical medicine had few innovations to heal the sick, and the effectiveness of cleanliness took decades to take hold in medical practice.

The quality of social life, in the form of education, was low. Some children remained illiterate, and much of the initiative began as Sunday Schools, an element which improved the quality of life and enriched the intern al life of a rising generation. In the matter of schooling as an expression of public policy, education in England and Wales came well after the development of National Schools in Ireland. Scotland had a system of education as a local custom long before the initiatives to the south.

**Table 3.1** Manchester, 1836: three occupational patterns of weekly expenditure[a]

| Item | Stoneman | | | | Laborer | | | | Weaver | | | |
|---|---|---|---|---|---|---|---|---|---|---|---|---|
| | £ | s | d | % | £ | s | d | % | £ | s | d | % |
| Rent | | 5 | 0 | 15.5 | | 3 | 5 | 18.3 | | 1 | 10 | 17.8 |
| Coal | | | | | | | 8 | 3.5 | | | 6 | 5.3 |
| Candles | | | 6 | 1.5 | | | 8 | 3.5 | | | 1.5 | 1.3 |
| Tobacco | | | 9 | 2.3 | | | | | | | | |
| Soap | | | 9 | 2.3 | | | 8 | 3.5 | | | 4 | 3.5 |
| Flour/bread | | 7 | 9 | 24.0 | | 3 | 9 | 2.0 | | 1 | 10 | 18.7 |
| Meat | | 6 | 3 | 19.4 | | 2 | 11 | 15.6 | | | 4.5 | 4 |
| Milk | | | | | | 2 | 0 | 10.7 | | | 10.5 | 9.3 |
| Potatoes | | 2 | | 6.2 | | | 6 | 2.6 | | | 5.5 | 4.9 |
| Tea | | 1 | 5.5 | 4.5 | | 9 | 2.5 | 4 | | | 6 | 5.3 |
| Sugar | | 1 | 8 | 5.2 | | 8 | 3.5 | | | | 5.5 | 4.9 |

[a]Neild (1841). System

**Table 3.2**  Child mortality by age, 1841–1855[a]

| Year | Live births | Mortality < 1 year | Mortality rate by age | | |
|---|---|---|---|---|---|
|  | Per 1000 | Per 1000 | 1–4 | 5–9 | 10–14 |
| 1841–1845 | 32.30 | 148 | – | 8.69 | 5.01 |
| 1846–1850 | 32.80 | 157 | – | 9.39 | 5.56 |
| 1851–1855 | 33.90 | 156 | – | 8.64 | 5.23 |

[a]Office of Population Censuses and Surveys (1985)

**Table 3.3**  VICQUAL index numbers at intervals of five years, 1815–1860 (Jordan, 1993a, b, c, d)

| Year | VICQUAL | Year | VICQUAL |
|---|---|---|---|
| 1815 | 95.73 | 1840 | 98.94 |
| 1820 | 92.05 | 1845 | 93.75 |
| 1825 | 98.76 | 1850 | 92.24 |
| 1830 | 98.05 | 1855 | 102.02 |
| 1835 | 96.76 | 1860 | 101.59 |

Within the representations of life in an era of empoverished quality commentators began to detect inferences for the overall society. Viewing factory workers they noted diminished physical condition and premature aging, as well as physical damage; the ravages of tuberculosis and other pulmonary conditions were widespread. The inference crystallized that each generation was a little weaker in a linear sense than the preceding. Mechanisms of inheritance were wildly misunderstood, so that the physical disorders, i.e. acquired characteristics, were thought likely to be inherited. One defective generation would produce another, and homo sapiens would regress. This misperception persisted well into the next century.

The degeneracy crisis among the Victorians was a public event in that merely encountering army recruits and factory workers revealed the parlous state of the peoples' health. At the end of the Victorian era the quality of physical life among young males had become a challenge to those seeking recruits for Queen Victoria's army. This passage closes with a numerical summary of social conditions at intervals of five years. The VICQUAL index numbers in Table 3.3 summarize five *Economic*, five *Social*, and, and four *Health* items; the criterion year is 1914. For annual index numbers see Jordan (1993a, b, c, d).

## 3.3   Victorian Female Criminals

In the several estimated ratings of individuals' quality of life the male role is indicated as advantageous; the reciprocal is that females, by virtue of their gender, were at a disadvantage.

This disability permeated Victorian society, and was evident in several ways. Public drunkenness was less likely to be tolerated by the policeman on his beat when the figure weaving down the street was a woman. Once in jail custodians might tolerate strong language from a man, but not when the offender was a woman.

Daughter to a woman with a long record Maria Adams aged seventeen years was sentenced to five years in prison for stealing clothes. That sentence followed several previous convictions for the same offence since she was fifteen. The crime was traditional among the poor, having been employed by a girl in the early stage of being hired in the mid-1 700s, by Elizabeth, the wife of diarist Samuel Pepys.

Apart from sentencing by gender the Law was harsh; stealing a watch guard and eight shillings in cash from Thomas Jebb brought down on Elizabeth Dyer a sentence of transportation to Tasmania for seven years. At age twenty six years she said goodbye to four children and her husband. Landed in Hobart Town she did not fare well, but she eventually settled down in Victoria, on the mainland, with a new husband, Edward Dyer, who lived a difficult life.

Sometimes convict life in Tasmania was alleviated by the presence of old ship-mates. In Tasmania Elizabeth Dyer had three friends from the convict ship, Emma Eugenia. Williams and Godfrey (2018) gave their names as, Susannah Wells, Eliza Conner, and Mary Leonard.

With the return of thousands of ex-soldiers and sailors from the Napoleonic wars the economy was insufficient to absorb them at a time when the need to produce goods and services for military use had declined sharply. At that time the economy had not yet begun the massive expansion, and proportional immiseration of the poor, which we see as a defining feature of the Victorian era. The social disintegration of the era resulted in an increase in crime; but that term, crime, tends to shimmer rather than appear in close focus because of the law's heavy hand.

That is, desperate people engaged in minor illegalities which an obsolete legal system deemed gross violations meriting legal punishments. In 1845, the era of the convicts considered here, Engels (1845) reported that a seventy two year-old man was sentenced to labor on the treadmill.

In the beginning years of the Long Peace the population outside London was mostly rural and poor. There were no police forces to prevent crime or arrest wrong doers. There was, however, a corpus of laws which retained the privileges of the wealthy, and punished offences. A crime meant an incident of some kind which had been identified, and then elaborated by recourse to laws, and prosecuted. Prosecution verbalized the offenses of earlier times, but many offenses never came to light. The village drunk might engage in offensive behavior, and the relations between men and women could be violent, but many incidents remained undetected. In one sense, our understanding of nineteenth century crime is an appreciation of prosecutions— events for which there was at least a nominal record. In another sense, there was much less crime because it went undetected and no one was called to account for his or her actions. Assaults on females as violations of male prerogatives by managers, and heads of households, went undetected, as in succeeding centuries. Restoration of pacific relations through divorce was rarely available.

On the other hand, there were behaviors which were judged harshly at the time. Such behaviors are, in today's morality, an episode needing little more than a reprimand, or a fine. Many were offenses involving property; picking pockets to extract silk kerchiefs was an entry level performance, and clothes might be stolen from clotheslines. On the other hand, crime on a large scale was also present. Many an engraved certificate memorializing purchase of mining or railway stock was worthless, but unloaded on the credulous. Earlier, there had been a steady encroachment on village lands traditionally available for grazing and growing crops. Local figures combining service as local justice of the peace with self-interest feathered their nests. The local populace—very often tenants—were powerless. An old verse recounted that,

The law will hang the man or woman who steals a goose from off the Common,

but lets the greater villain loose who steals the Common from under the goose.

That piece of doggerel catches the differing rates of social change; the couplet contrasts sharp rural practices against the background of law unimproved for generations.

In the presence of social tension of many kinds resort to physical violence was likely, and also undetectable. Such identification presumed a social order in which protection of persons and property was deliberate across communities. Not until Sir Robert Peel organized a formal force of for law enforcement policemen would pursuit of crime present the outline of personnel and formal roles with which we are broadly familiar with today. However, the introduction caused some Britons to bristle at the introduction of a semi- military force into the fabric of society. A part of the change in outlook was a reluctance to introduce Chadwick-like records as a routine procedure, but Victorian crime statistics are scarce until the later decades of the nineteenth century.

In passing it is useful to recall the combination of violence and politics. An assassin failed in an attempt to assassinate Queen Victoria while she was riding in her carriage. Later, the Irish Fenian movement resorted to violence in order to achieve political ends.

One of the contributions to reducing crime was the construction of new prisons. Within them new, but hopeless systems, were introduced. The treadmill and solitary confinement were new modes of molding behavior and forms of punishment.

Jeremy Bentham's *Panopticon* was a revolutionary design which enabled a prison warden to see along several corridors which spread out fanwise from a central observation site. Assignment to a convict ship was a welcome alternative to dispatch to a *hulk*, an abandoned, dismasted warship. Some transported felons came from hulks.

In the long run it seemed easier, less complicated, and cheaper to simply dispatch felons to Australia; the cost per head was about £15. On that premise, men, women, and children were sent on the long voyage to the southern ocean. The goal was merely to purge the body-politic of its corrosive members with np provision for return after a sentence had been served. It may be noted that in the earliest passages various combinations of crew, marines, men, women and children were tried until less tempestuous combinations were devised. It was a premise of the times that criminality was a moral failure. In the earliest voyages morality was set back to a considerable degree by arrangements in the sailing vessels. The State failed to provide sufficient supplies for the early voyages, and the mixing of the genders created a self-fulfilling prophecy of corrupted rather than enhanced morality.

## 3.4 Australia

With the loss of access to much of North America formalized though the Treaty of Paris the surrender of British forces at Yorktown in 1781 closed the scarcely explored continent to the British government as a place to dump felons. Over the next several years Whitehall chose the scarcely understood continent, Australia, as a penal colony. Known from the explorations of Dutch voyagers, and more focally that of Captain James Cook, Australia was far enough away to act as a banishment for criminals expelled from the British Isles. Unlike North America, the indigenous population was small and, in the case of Tasmania to the south, quickly suppressed or killed. To the southeast of Australia, New Zealand's Polynesian population was sophisticated, but coercion and shrewd negotiating (e.g.) the Treaty of Waitangi, facilitated settlement by British immigrants. Whether a secondary goal, or not, Whitehall's attention to Australia and New Zealand spread the color red on maps of the south-east Pacific.

The place to which the First Fleet of ships transporting convicts sailed in 1788, unlike the two major islands of New Zealand, was a continent. Composed of a large central desert surrounded, for the most part, by temperate lands, Australia subsequently revealed valuable minerals, and an array of curious mammals, of which the Kangaroo is the most obvious member. The indigenous people were spread thinly living a life complicated by rituals and understandings alien to the new settlers; the arrival of the steel axe was a utilitarian step to settlers, but it provoked cultural complications for the indigenous folk. By virtue of its distance and the relevant ignorance of London policy makers Australia became a cheap alternative to building prisons and hiring and training men (and later women) to enforce the expanding body of criminal laws.

## 3.5 The First Fleet

From several parts of the British mainland prisoners sentenced to transportation for petty and for major crimes were dispatched from their home towns and hamlets. Many had been found guilty of offenses we consider petty and punish with a reprimand—if even prosecuted. Today's equivalent might be a parking meter violation.

At the time, however, the law came down heavily on stealing a sheep, or offering a remark deemed an impertinence by a powerful figure. On the other hand, it would have required an offence on a largish scale where smuggling was sanctioned by local custom, and the local JP was suspected of enjoying French brandy as well as anyone else. In some cases, a jury reduced the value of stolen or smuggled goods to reduce proven or admitted guilt below the level of capital punishment. Whatever the individual case histories many prisoners were brought to ships at anchor off the Isle of Wight on England's south coast.

Under the command of Captain Arthur Phillips, according to Preston (2017), there gathered a fleet of eleven ships, seaworthy but not large, to receive convicts. The size of these vessels may be gauged by the width or beam of the largest ship, HMS *Alexander*, which was thirty one feet (Preston, 2017). Inference of an appalling quality of life at sea for convicts is easy to imagine, as ships rolled and pitched amidst the waves of the south Atlantic, and the summer heat of the endless Indian Ocean.

Aboard convict ships, (and several vessels will be addressed shortly) the quality of life for convicts was structured physically by the shortage of space. In addition to the narrow beam there was the restricted height between decks. The lack of portholes open to daylight, fresh air, and cleansing winds confined any disease organisms to the space 'tween-decks'. As with the situation of emigrants in Chap. 2, sailing the Atlantic a ship's doctor—if there was one—could detect gross illness as passengers came aboard, and indents (ships' records) were filled out, but latent diseases in people not yet showing gross symptoms would infect those who came aboard free of disease. Whatever personal quality of life was brought on board by a passenger was compromised by the health of others, and the temporary culture generated on the long voyage.

The quality of psychological life probably included the anxious and bewildered among those felons so deemed by the law, but in actuality merely people who succumbed to an impulse. At the other extreme were psychopathic criminals ending a life of crime and casting around for things to steal and passengers to exploit. The latter would include Marine guards and the crew. In the case of females, a pretty smile and a pleasant manner might lead to acquiring a patron and privileges. Having served on the convict ship, *Kains*, Dr. Thomas Clarke recalled "...*conversation with each other most abandoned, without feeling or shame*" (Bateson, 1974) (Table 3.4).

Given the length of the voyage and the months of physical proximity, the end of the voyage, regardless of the personal outcome, would have been a great relief. For some, relief was in the form of death, since the circumstances of a convict voyage were extreme, and exodus in the form of a sack with weights and a few words from a chaplain, or the Captain, would have seen the corpse over the side into Davy Jones' Locker, as weather permitted. However, most female convicts survived, and were put ashore, after which the crew prepared the ship for the return voyage.

At the time, Hobart Town had about seven thousand inhabitants, and the *Harmony* women would have found work as domestic servants. Not all would have been suitable since for many the sentence of transportation beyond the seas came about after several

**Table 3.4** Population of Australia, in thousands, 1821–1891, by decade

| Decade | 1821 | 1831 | 1841 | 1851 | 1861 | 1871 | 1881 | 1891 |
|---|---|---|---|---|---|---|---|---|
| Thousands | 39 | 76 | 221 | 438 | 1168 | 1668 | 1668 | 2250 |

*Source* Carrier and Jeffery (1953)

prior convictions. Also, some of the women probably were alcoholics, and were likely to fall back into patterns of alcoholism. That condition by itself would have brought them to the attention of the Tasmanian authorities and led to a variety of consequences. Women who were working as servants would have been discharged, and, if fortunate, might have been assisted by church-based philanthropy (Fig. 3.2).

Marriage seems to have been rare, recalling that the stigma of their conviction did not erode, as it did for male convicts. Around 1830, values limited females to modest roles in English-speaking society. It seems fair to summarize the fate of the landed female convicts as one of limited opportunities as they lived out their sentences of banishment to the Antipodes. Virtually all of them died in Tasmania, since return to the British Isles was expensive, and could only have arisen as an opportunity after their several years of banishment had ended.

By the 1840s The young Victoria had been Queen for several years, and had married Albert in 1840. The country was at peace. Literacy within the population was substantial, and growing. However, social tensions were rising and would lead in 1838 to the People's Charter. In the revolutionary year 1848, a meeting was planned for Kennington Common, but it rained and the meeting fizzled; the petition was delivered by horse-powered cab, and the reform impulse failed. Tuberculosis was a constant menace within the population and it took the lives of several of the children of the Yorkshire vicar, the Rev, Patrick Bronte. The factory towns expanded with a corresponding degree of social disorganization; abuse of alcohol was a recognized problem, and crime was another. Unlike the *Harmony* women of 1829, the men of the *John Renwick* and the *John Brewer* considered in this Chapter were mostly born in the Midlands, and a modest ten percent were born in London. Place of birth was not necessarily the place of the crime leading to transportation, although the population was fairly settled, but young people walked to find work, when necessary.

Another contrast with female convicts was the wider range of claimed occupations. about two thirds claimed prior skilled urban occupations. That may have been true, but such skills seem unlikely to pre-dispose men to a life of crime. An alternative

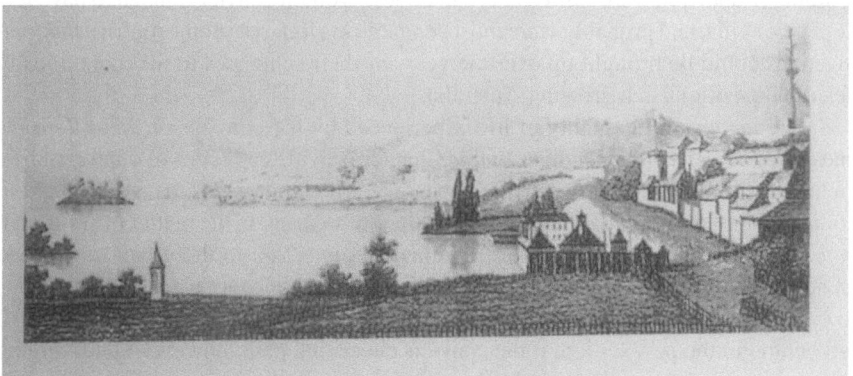

**Fig. 3.2**  A view of Point Puer

hypothesis is that the convicts used the occasion of being recorded in the indents as a way to predispose hiring officials in Hobart to see them favorably, and so avoid hard physical labor.

The ranks of convicts occasionally included men with middle class backgrounds, an example being a man who stole books for his own use from a college library. another man, one whose social stratum was privileged was William Smith O'Brien, an Irish politician well-connected within the Anglo-Irish Establishment. In 1828 Smith O'Brien entered Parliament and became well known among the landed gentry. Among the *John Brewer* and *John Renwick* convicts were men in late adolescence; for them nomination of an occupation for the indent probably was not thought through, and may have set them down as unskilled laborers. The youngest convict, Patrick Dempsey, stood a very modest four feet and two inches, and was ten years old. His indent recorded his brown hair, blue eyes, and fresh complexion. Sending a ten-year old Londoner to Australia was probably intended by the sentencing magistrate as an act of kindness offering the hope of a fresh start. On the other hand, we can only speculate about the tricks he could have picked up in the company of career criminals.

Tasmania. Most convicts survived the long voyage to the island south of the Australian mainland. However, their custodians were motivated by self-interest; only with delivery of convicts physically equipped to work would contracted fees be paid by the government in London.

Traffic across the vast ocean was brisk in the early 1840s. Bateson (1974) identified twenty four transports delivering their human cargo to Hobart Town in 1843, and another eighteen in 1842. Hobart, to use the current name, received 4643 males in 1842. (Females in that year amounted to 476 persons). The practice of expelling felons from Britain to Australia did not end until 1868, a period of 81 years. As with American colonists the 1770s, and Canadians in the early twentieth century, public opinion did not favor receipt of people who were not tolerated at home. Also, British public opinion turned against exiling convicts to the far reaches of the globe.

Examining data from the two ships is productive in the matter of useful skills. About half of the convicts of 1842–43 appear to have been unskilled urbanites, while a similar proportion were skilled at urban trades. Women convicts tended to have few domestic skills, and probably were most vendable in Hobart as domestic servants, and juveniles could be brought up over the years of their sentences to fill economically desirable positions in a growing Australia.

In the matter of the quality of life experienced by the convicts on *John Renwick* and *John Brewer* two appendices to this Chapter provide estimates of quality of life. Gender favored males in the nineteenth century, which put males in a good position, compared to females, after they had served their sentences. In the matter of skills men who, prior to transportation to Australia had a connection to the urban trades, had an advantage. A single state, rather than being married, meant few or no dependents to provide for. Prior convictions were a shared state among convicts, and could be left behind in the new setting, if the convicts chose that path; however, status among convicts probably depended on the degree of outrage their crimes elicited. Few had assets to capitalize on, conserve, or pre-conviction skills. It is hard to see any money getting from England to Tasmania via the ship-born experience.

On the other hand, what few assets brought onto ships might wax or wane as games of chance permitted. Being English-speaking was the common experience, although rural speakers of Gaelic probably fitted in fairly quickly. The pre-conviction health of convicts probably was poor, and some probably went on board carrying infectious organisms. On the other hand, deaths at sea were uncommon. The voyage itself was stressful access the fresh air often meant time on deck in chains. Hobart Town itself was an accessible port, providing job opportunities, and access to other towns. Food at hand on the voyage was restricted to whatever the ships' owners provided. Some convict ships had officially recognized physicians. However, anyone with simple skills in the tradition of barber-surgeons, e.g. pulling teeth, would have been put to work. The vessels which transported convicts appear to have been built well. John Brewer was built at Redbridge in 1811, and was young for the era.

It is likely that some convict ships also conveyed colonists to Colombia in South America. A Scottish contingent which included many young persons emigrated in1827. For persons arriving in Tasmania, a link to kith and kin, including fellow convicts, would have been a source of support in several way. Tasmania, for the ex-convict offered opportunities for the free men to acquire property. Tasmania had a vigorous lumber business. Hobart Town was a vigorous and growing place, having been a useful urban settlement of several thousand people for several years. Finally, once a convict had been formally discharged from his sentence, probably having been a ticket-of leave man towards the end, such a person was free, and most chose to stay in Tasmania or the other flourishing settlements of the Antipodes.

## 3.6   The Ship, *Harmony*

In 1828 the convict ship, *Harmony* left the south coast of England as the gales of Autumn ushered in a change of season. Ahead lay a voyage of thirteen thousand miles in a cockleshell of a vessel sent out to enter the stormy Atlantic. Beyond the Cape of Good Hope,—an irony probably not lost on the passengers who would at a later date reflect on the irony of the ship's name. The longest and most isolated leg of the voyage was the long distance from South Africa to Tasmania—at the time, still known as Van Diemen's Land. A course set too far south in order to catch the westerly winds known and feared by sailors as The Roaring Forties; after one hundred and twenty three days at sea, their prospect would have lifted the spirits of *Harmony*'s passengers, despite a revived uncertainty shaping their psychological outlook.

It may be noted that not every passenger on a convict ship came from the lower levels of society. The would-be revolutionary figure in Ireland, William Smith O'Brien, was caught at the early stage of his would-be insurrection; tolerant of his amateurism and his respectability he was not executed but banished to Australia. His transit was under benign ship conditions, and in Australia he lived in a cottage. Smith O'Brien ended his days back in Ireland quite purged of any thoughts of insurrection.

On 14 January, 1829, *Harmony* dropped anchor in Hobart Town, under Captain Bennet Ireland. Ten years earlier, The Penny Magazine, in 1832, described Hobart Town:

> The town stands upon gently rising ground, and covers more than a square mile. Its streets are wide, and intersect each other at right angles. it contains several government buildings, a parish church, and other places of worship, a government school for the poor, and several Sunday schools...Hobart Town possesses a distillery, two timber mills...the population is above seven thousand. (Jordan, 1993a, b, c, d)

The ship *Harmony* was comparatively new being a mere ten years in service after being built in St. Johns, Newfoundland and she served as a convict ship more than once. The quality of thought leading to the voyage of *Harmony* was mixed. On the one hand were the observations of Mr. Bennet Ireland, an experienced mariner while, on the other, there were other officials with, apparently, little or no grasp of what a voyage to the south seas entailed. in particular, there was the composition of the felons to be transported—an aggregate of one hundred females in a bimodal distribution of ages, brought together at the Downs off the coast of Kent. The women came from a variety of backgrounds, and most had been domestics; an exception was Elizabeth Mills from Houndley Green, listed as a potter. Seventeen of the women had a shared background in London. No less unique in background were sixteen women whose origins were in Ireland, and from the largely Catholic hinterlands beyond Dublin. They shared cultural elements, and it seems likely that some of them spoke little English. The fourteen women from Scotland, north of the Glasgow—Edinburgh connection would have had difficulty speaking easily, and being understood. Their relationship with the other women would have been strained until experiences of the voyage created a shared culture of misery and low expectations. The typical *Harmony* woman was in her mid-twenties, and in view of the era's life expectancy, probably could anticipate fifteen or more years left in her life cycle. Across those years, the older *Harmony* women could reflect on family members left behind; that is, a few were married, and left husbands, children and, possibly, grandchildren behind.

The other miscalculation by the planners of the 1829 voyage was the presence of guards—frequently volunteering Marines discovering a way to emigrate. Some took wives and children, while others were hitherto unattached. The married men probably felt a hope of success orientation in their inner contemplations. Such a hope, like that of Dickens' Wilkins McCawber, could be an effective motivator from which to start a new life.

To be Captain of such a complement, as was the role of Captain Ireland, was to assume a very difficult role. His control of the women was formally defined. He may not flog a woman, but he could shave her head. The Old Adam was a supernumerary on such a voyage. During the four-month voyage, the formality of inter-personal relations would have eroded, and unattached males probably used their superior status to advantage. On a voyage of several months attachments developed, and pregnancies would have occurred. The ship's indents contain notes entered by the doctor, William Clifford; he noted that Catherine parsons had a "long scar on her forehead over right eye," Elizabeth Smith, formerly a cook, was nearly blind in her right eye, and Elizabeth Miller had an unspecified speech defect.

As the voyage of the Harmony approached its end the convict women were issued serge petticoats, a pair of shifts, a cap, stockings, and a pair of shoes. A woman with domestic skills might have knitted caps and other articles of clothing to sell in Hobart Town. However, such a tranquil soul seems to have been an exception in view of the words of evaluation recorded by Surgeon Thomas Clarke on the quality of life experienced on the ship *Kain* transporting female convicts:

> If there ever was a hell afloat it must have been in the shape of a female convict ship— quarrelling, fighting, thieving, from a mere spirit of devilisness, destroying in private each other's property, conversations with each other most abandoned, without feeling or shame. Bateson (1974)

## 3.7  Tasmania

Generally speaking convicts on transport ships reached their destinations alive; deaths occurred and were dealt with expeditiously. Arriving at their destinations was due, in part, to the system's set of terms which guided ship-board practices. After word had been received in London of a successful voyage the contractors' bill was paid; The ship's physician received ten shillings and sixpence for each convict arriving in good health; that is, fit after an assessment by the local Superintendent of Convicts. He had authority to assign men to tasks for which they claimed competence. Relevant were occupations for which there was known demand. In the case of the two ships considered here trades among the convicts for which there was a known demand in Tasmania were: brickmaker, carpenter, mason, harness maker, and "engineer"—the latter probably anyone with experience with machinery. A man who had worked in a factory around machines of any kind might well have found useful employment. In Tasmania, convicts were not herded into prisons and could make their own future.

Among the transported men there were few who really grasped where they were. Among the convicts on the Australian mainland were a few who believed that China was a little to the north, and who fled, only to disappear for good in the "great outback."

Among the landed convicts were men to whom violence was familiar, and disturbances led to creation of a prison within a prison. A separate prison was established at distant Norfolk Island for prisoners in Australia who broke local laws. In contrast, there were transported convicts who prospered in their Asian setting. A reality was that very few, perhaps six percent of transported convicts, returned to the British Isles. An irony is that that the Canadian, Francis X. Prieur, one of those who returned to Canada, became the Minister for prisons.

Others who chose to remain (merely for lack of opportunity, in some cases,) took advantage of the Ticket-of-leave system which extended opportunities for the already fairly mobile transportees. Two Appendices summarize my estimate of the quality of life experienced by Australia's new residents.

## 3.8   The *Lord Goderich* and the *Frances Charlotte*

On a weekday in the Lancashire mill town, Preston, The Magistrate was dealing in his usual stern, but privately sympathetic manner, with a procession of local scoundrels. Most of the charges were thefts of property, and he dispatched the miscreants to prison, restitution, fines, or sent them on their way. After disposing of one case, a juvenile, one can imagine that the Magistrate told the Clerk of the Court to summon the next case. "There he is," mumbled the Clerk." I see no one" observed the Magistrate. "Let's get on with the Court's business "he added sharply.

In fact the accused was there. Being perhaps four feet tall a real lad from the rough streets of Preston, Dominick Rafferty, stood behind the bar of the Dock, but was invisible. Dominick, who could not see over the front of the Dock, was charged with stealing nine penny coins. Shocked when the child was pointed out to him the magistrate declared a recess in the proceedings. Turning to his Clerk he pointed out for all present to hear, that the legal system was inflexible, and quite inappropriate to deal with the small child before him. In the end, after consultation he assigned the criminal to the care of a local Methodist charity. In another case heard in London an eight-year old girl who stole goods valued at five shillings and sixpence was sentenced to six months in jail.

The law at mid-century was an aggregate of accrued elements dating back for centuries. It presumed that all charged persons were similar when arraigned, and that courts would treat all persons similarly; the figure of justice was blind—and also tone deaf in the matter of children. Reformers were vocal but Parliament was slow to move beyond legal precedents.

At Westminster, Lord Shaftesbury emerged as "The Children's Friend," and for the popular press the artist John Leech presented to the public in 1841 his Children of the Mobility sketches, a series of drawings intended to introduce the middle class to the "Mobility," the opposite of the privileged *Nobility,* that is, the children of the urban poor.

However, in the year of Leech's sketches boys were still placed on the sailing ship *Lord Goderich* (1841) for the long voyage to Tasmania. That action was similar to the voyage, a decade before, of the *Frances Charlotte* (1832), on her first assignment as a convict ship. In this chapter the experiences of both ships are combined; the passage of a decade brought only slight changes to a fundamentally appalling procedure. An innovation was the assignment of boys to Parkhurst Prison where strict discipline was expected to remediate the moral failure which had brought them into the healing embrace of the prison system. The latter was operated on the premise that young criminals were destined to become old criminals, and potentially gallows-bound.

Among the combined total of three hundred and six boys (the separate ships' numbers being quite similar) there were a few men in their twenties; William Sharpe from Leeds, and William Draker were both thirteen years old. Inspecting boys at Parkhurst, the reformer, James Kay-Shuttleworth found them to be "…deficient in physical organization;" at the time, juvenile delinquents were short, like Preston's Dominick Rafferty, and were visible evidence of an impending degeneracy in the national population. Juvenile delinquents in the Victorian years frequently bore tattoos as a sign of criminal identity. Placed in the flesh between thumb and the palm of the hand the tattoo could be concealed and revealed at will.

We know little of the fate of the boys landed at Hobart Town; however, it is generally known that second generation immigrants to Australia have been taller and healthier than their parents. However, all that Tasmania had to offer was the juvenile colony outside Hobart known as Point Puer (*puer* meaning boy). Close to Port Arthur on a narrow strip of land this colony intended to segregate youthful offenders operated for about fifteen years, closing in 1649; technically, it was sponsored by the prison at Port Arthur. Over the course of its active service Point Puer provided strict control, but as an assembly of several hundred young males, all of whom had at least a minimal reason for transportation, it created its own subculture. Bullying, extortion and other forms of exploitation probably undid the moral and vocational benefits its managers sought.

The fundamental flaw in the practice of transportation was that it sent juveniles across the world; it had flourished briefly in seventeenth century London when children living on the streets were rounded up and shipped to the North American colonies. However, as a school for crime-prone young males segregation overseas of the young from mature criminals was a sound idea. Unfortunately, British society generally subscribed to the idea that reform was a rare event, and that physical punishment was the modality for inducing moral reform and so reducing crime. Put simply, the goal was to get rid of trouble in the form of child crime. Mitigating that principle was the four-month voyage with adult criminals, in many cases. The opening of Parkhurst Prison on the Isle of Wight was a forward step in prison reform. In contrast, Point Puer was a failure.

Militating against success were the values of the Victorian era. Morality was strictly held. Given the evils of the day, alcoholism, abusive factory management, and the conviction that the formation of personal virtue meant physical coercion of the young, reform was an uphill battle. The Chartist movement at mid-century showed that peaceful political-social movements required a broader, deeper base than the population was willing to support. The Establishment tentatively corrected society at the margins, but reform was left to high-minded people whose social innovations merely ameliorated conditions. Not until the political reforms of the 1860 s, three decades after the great Reform law of 1832, did power shift towards ordinary, that is to say, poor people.

Formation of labor unions moved towards political reform, and public recognition of the egalitarian values of society's majority. Educational reform and innovation came slowly, and it was in Ireland that innovation came first, creating a sense that schooling was a tool for modernization. The modernizing Irish child became an object of attention, if only on grounds of fiscal conservatism. But children moved from the wings to center stage steadily.

On that premise, rounding up young males and then shipping them thirteen thousand miles, far from family, and whatever social context they knew, deprived them of a social context within which they could be socialized to advantage.

Still there persisted the idea that children were hard to recover from social risks. But, at Point Puer, the mentors were themselves nominally rehabilitated criminals. Such role models were uncertain agents of change in the lives of young males. Nothing had been learned from the seventeenth century practice of shipping young males, and some females, to North America under the guise of acquiring vocational skills.

Probably most pernicious was the ideology that the State had authority to expel its citizens, male, female, and children out of the country. The social contract on which the country was run was a sham, although the fine points of social theorizing were met with indifference as conservative reformers, the Shuttleworth brothers, Mary Carpenter, Lord Shaftesbury, and later Thomas Barnardo and Robert Baden-Powell among others, sought to salvage youngsters living at social risk for a range of adverse outcomes to childhood. The radical reformers sought revolutionary changes, and were willing to use violence to that end. The data amassed in anchester's cotton spinning mills by Friedrich Engels called for an end to the prevailing social horizons of the British people. Such radicalism was unacceptable at all levels of British society. Goaded by the words of "The Childrens' Friend," Lord Shaftesbury, Establishment people found their Evangelical enthusiasms aroused, and legal updating began its long journey through the consciences of the privileged.

In summary, the two "ships of clever lads," experienced an average to poor quality of life before a criminal act. The harsh legal system of the Victorian era, led to transportation beyond the seas to Hobart, Tasmania, in the Great Southern Ocean. They then travelled under stern conditions for about four months in transit to Tasmania. At Hobart, the youngsters were displayed to possible employers as a work force, a role that their under-developed physiques restricted to tasks requiring little strength. Their quality of life in Tasmania is undocumented, but we may infer that it was poor. Point Puer probably increased juveniles' hostility to authority figures, setting up a tension with would-be employers. The archaism of the law in the early years of Queen Victoria's era was evident in the insensitivity to children as a special group. The reality of their situation was recognized by individual magistrates, but they were bound to invoke the law conservatively—until conscience dictated another course.

We now turn to providing a sense of the quality of life experienced by the juveniles sent to Hobart, Tasmania early in the reign of Queen Victoria using the schema of eighteen topics previously employed in Chap. 2.

Gender, even the gender of the young was important in Victorian society. The young males expelled to Tasmania were conscious of their masculinity, a vector of maturity inculcating the culture of crime in Victorian days. Older boys were models for the younger group, and past criminal achievements were listened to attentively. Tricks of the trade were passed around, and the innovation of Point Puer showed its vulnerability to omission of empirical data in the process of forming public policy in Whitehall, and in the spirited debates at Westminster. Indeed, as late as the middle years of the twentieth century, public figures were bemoaning the surges of information swamping the polished tones of men in public life whose glittering generalities tended to be merely rhetorical devices.

# Appendix 1: Numerical Estimate of Adult Immigrants to Australia, Quality of Life

| Domain | Rating | | | | |
|---|---|---|---|---|---|
| | −2 | −1 | 0 | +1 | +2 |
| Gender (M) | | | | | ☺ |
| Skills | | | ○ | | |
| Single | | | | ☺ | |
| Convicted | | ☹ | | | |
| Assets | | | | | ☺ |
| English-speaking | | | | ☺ | |
| Health | | | ○ | | |
| Weather | | | ○ | | |
| Nearby port | | | | ☺ | |
| Food at hand | | | | | ☺ |
| Barber/surgeon | | | | | ☺ |
| Sturdy vessel | | | | | ☺ |
| Kith and kin | | | | | ☺ |
| Property | | | ○ | | |
| Urban settlement | | | | | ☺ |
| *Indenture* | | | | | |
| – Discharged | | | | | ☺ |
| – Fled | | | | ☺ | |
| – Cheated | ☹ | | | | |

# Appendix 2: Numerical Estimate of Young Male Convicts to Australia, Quality of Life

| Domain | Rating | | | | |
|---|---|---|---|---|---|
| | −2 | −1 | 0 | +1 | +2 |
| Gender (M) | | | | | ☺ |
| Skills | | | ○ | | |

(continued)

(continued)

| Domain | Rating | | | | |
|---|---|---|---|---|---|
| Single | | | | ☺ | |
| Convicted | | ☹ | | | |
| Assets | | | | | ☺ |
| English-speaking | | | | ☺ | |
| Health | | | ○ | | |
| Weather | | | ○ | | |
| Nearby port | | | | ☺ | |
| Food at hand | | | | | ☺ |
| Barber/surgeon | | | | | ☺ |
| Sturdy vessel | | | | | ☺ |
| Kith and kin | | | | | ☺ |
| Property | | | ○ | | |
| Urban settlement | | | | | ☺ |
| *Indenture* | | | | | |
| – Discharged | | | | | ☺ |
| – Fled | | | | ☺ | |
| – Cheated | | | | ☹ | |

# References

Bateson, C. C. (1974). *The convict ships 1787–1868*. Wellington: Reed.

Carrier, N. H., & Jeffery, J. R. (1953). *External migration: A study of the available statistics 1815–1950*. London: Her Majesty's Stationery Office.

Engels, F. (1845). *The condition of the working class in England*. Moscow: Progress.

Jordan, T. E. (1993a). Estimating the quality of life for children around the world: NICQL—92. *Social Indicators Research, 30,* 17–38.

Jordan, T. E. (1993b). *The degeneracy crisis and Victorian youth*. Albany, NY: SUNY Press.

Jordan, T. E. (1993c). "*Stay and starve or go and prosper!*" Juvenile emigration from Great Britain in the nineteenth century. *Social Science History, 9,* 145–166.

Jordan, T. E. (1993d). "L'Homme Moyen:" Estimating the quality of life for British adults, 1815–1914. *Social Indicators Research, 29,* 183–203.

Neild, W. (1841). Comparative statement of the income and expenditure of certain families of the working class in Manchester and Dukinfield, 1836 and 1841. *Journal of the Royal Statistical Society, 4,* 320–324.

Office of Population Censuses and Surveys. (1985). Mortality statistics. Social tables. Series DH1, no. 15. London: Her Majesty's Stationery Office.

Preston, D. (2017). *Paradise in chains*. New York, NY: Bloomsbury.

Williams, L., & Godfrey, B. (2018). *Criminal women: Researching the lives of female criminals in Britain and Australia*. Barnsley (UK): Pen and Sword.

# Chapter 4
# The Quality of Internal Life

**Abstract** So far, in this consideration of quality of life, the focus has been on the social nature of people. Two groups have been considered using their numeric nature, that is, the accretion of information from more than one person, to infer the quality of life in the age of sailing ships. We now turn to internal aspects of the human experience in order to recognize the subjective aspect of quality of life.

**Keywords** Migration · The self · Motivation · Life cycle · Ireland · Modernism · Comparisons

People have an internal life, a consciousness of the world and the people with whom they interact. The internal life consists of experiences, memories, images, and phantasies which are dealt with rationally and irrationally. This array of events is organized within the brain and gives rise to a sense of self, a perception that a singularity of consciousness exists with a sense of continuity. This last construct evolves during the course of a temporal unit-the 24-h day into the sleep mode in which contents are re-organized in what we call dreams. In that state the sense of a personal identity, the self, persists but on a less rational basis.

## 4.1   The Self

The self is perceived and is amenable to consideration as experiencing degrees of quality, i.e. internal quality of life (Of course, here we presume normality for purposes of discussion.). Across the life-span, the self experiences degrees of quality within the nexus of living; inconsistency and ambiguity are lived with as people cope with the realities of daily life. Across such modalities the self adjusts to differing states of being and responds to drives or motives.

The latter are perceived only partially, originating sometimes from constitutional elements of human nature in some cases. Routinely, the self defends itself from unpleasant components, or copes with the demands of an element of the self, conscience. In her study of stress in the lives of children Werner (1989) found that some young people have a greater intrinsic tolerance for social stress than other young people. This trait appears to be due to other than socialization. Of course, such an opaque trait has no apparent source, but it defends the self in times of stress. On the other hand, there are theorists who believe that identity is an illusion, and is an unprofitable construct (see Holmes, 2019).

Self emerges from the cellular levels of the brain in processes yet to be understood. Self is generally considered dynamic, interacting with the senses, with perceived social reality, and the contents of' memory. On the other hand, there are theorists who believe that identity is an illusion (Holmes, 2019). One outcome of human development, autonomous or accultured, is the vital role of motives. They are forces which, sometimes irrationally and often unperceived, determine overt action.

## 4.2   Motivation

Maslow (1954) saw motives in a hierarchy which was preserving and complex. Maslow saw as a basic motive survival of the individual; his collation of motives is as follows:

Basic is the preservation of the body in which Physiological Needs prevail.

Above that level is the need to be Safe.

With that condition satisfied there arise Emotional-Social considerations.

Which precipitate the need for Esteem,

and still higher is the pursuit of Self-Actualization.

Maslow's schema is often presented as a triangle with Physiological Needs as the base, and *Self-Actualization* as the apex.

A motive influencing human outcomes in any generation (e.g. immigrants and young soldiers) is the drive to achieve (de Charms, 1968). The Achievement Motive brings structure to the tasks of life and consists of competition with a standard of excellence. This motive requires the self to strive towards a high level of quality in whatever task is deemed important; not every task is valued so highly, and striving for quality has produced outstanding achievements in several fields of human endeavor.

The range of human motives is wide, and it is influenced by the ethos of the times. Among seventeenth century Europeans Christianity generated widely a zeal for religious enthusiasms. People we know today as Puritans fled what they considered oppression by the established Anglican church: they left East Anglia (for the most part) for Holland, and then migrated to the New World. Of course, not everyone was so motivated, and the folk addressed in Chap. 2 tended to have material reasons for their hegira. Evans (2017) found motives in ordinary peoples' lives: some sought a better life and opportunity, while others experienced economic distress when, for example, fluctuations in the wool trade led to loss of income and unemployment. Still others migrated to London from the provinces but found little or no economic security, and then moved on to the New World; for a discussion of how people became emigrants see Evans (2017). Wareing's (2017) account of "Indentured Migration and the Servant Trade ..." traced the migration of English people to the Chesapeake and nearby colonies. Bailyn's earlier work details the forces at work on the east coast of the unexplored continent (Bailyn, 1985, 2012).

## 4.3   Migration

Seventeenth century migrants. Chapter 2's immigrants are opaque to analysis in many ways: they rarely left traces of their struggles which frequently ended in early death— by current standards. However, there are challenges which every generation faces, and they arise in the search to define oneself. Immigrants to the Chesapeake, while still living in the Home Counties of southern England, for the most part (Evans, 2017), experienced a disturbance of the self—itself the basis for the decision to migrate. The degree of insecurity probably lowered mood and raised anxiety. Risk-taking seemed dangerous, but the absence of security narrowed the choices. At the same time it seems likely that whatever sense of personal integrity prevailed honesty, charity, piety, and independence, etc. would permeate the self and protect the sense of worth, to a degree, across the phases of migration.

To most emigrants the coastal ports were novel and the sea voyage was a first-time experience: it required considerable discomfort and the salience of Maslow's Physiological Needs. For Mistress Janet Shaw her experience of green waves flooding her cabin elevated mere survival to a priority. On arrival in the New World, depending on the contractual circumstance, Immigrants' sense of self required reorientation; they were lessened in self-worth and mood by their changed social status. Children born in the colonies were not stigmatized by the immigrant status of their parent.

Exposure to harsh working conditions was the immediate fate of felons. Over time that situation evolved and African slave labor replaced English convict labor. Little or no information appears to exist about the sense of self experienced by African slaves as their numbers grew across the seventeenth century. After 1776 "beyond the seas ... " remained an attractive theme for judicial authorities in Britain (Ekirch, 2011), and devious schemes to export felons emerged. South Africa and, later, Australia became places to exile felons.

Returning to the experience of Richard Frethorne we can only speculate about the years after his letters intended to release him from his indenture, and so facilitate his emancipation. Having survived the voyage to Virginia he may have exhausted his quantum of good luck, and perished at a fairly young age. It seems unlikely that he would have endured his circumstances and, after a specified number of years, received the emoluments provided for in his articles of indenture. Those benefits were legally binding, but enforcement in Virginia was far from certain except where county courts were well established. The situation in Martin's Hundred was not promising. Figure 4.1 provides a four-stage suggestion of factors which stimulate the internal processing of sensory inputs. At these four stages the self-sifts and re-arranges materials; the outcome is a mental state of varying degrees by stage. The four young women who sailed to Tasmania on the convict ship *Emma Eugenia* were already socialized into social class expectations of their roles as women, and subsequently as felons. As the convict ship neared Hobart Town there remained the question of what the immediacy of arrival and its transitions would generate.

Some of the four women might have been stripped of their crime-related outlooks (weltanschauung) and acquired sense that the future was open-ended. In that state, a hope-of-success motivation might spur them to good outcomes in their new lives. On the other hand, the miserable conditions on the *Emma Eugenia* persisted for several

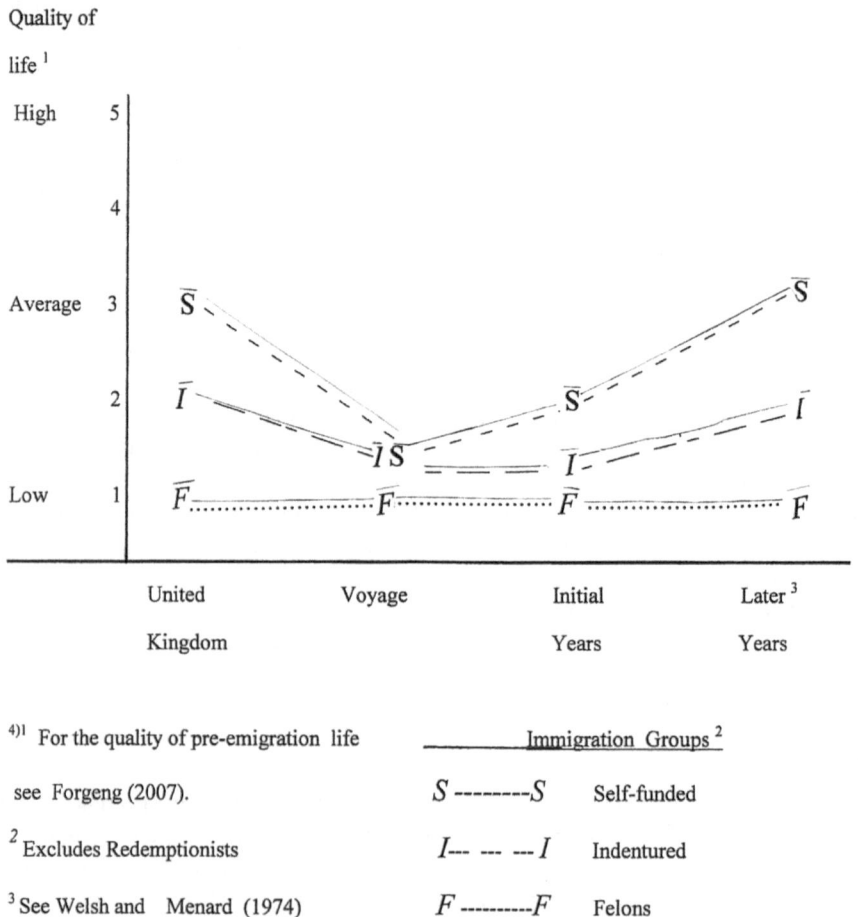

**Fig. 4.1** Estimated quality of life[1]—the immigrant life cycle to America

months; depression and an increased fear-of-failure were equally likely outcomes as the young women—Elizabeth Dyer, Susannah Wells, Eliza Conner, and Mary Leonard—stepped ashore onto dry land after months of rolling waves and a sense of the profound isolation which the south Atlantic Ocean and the endless Indian Ocean echoed.

Among those young women, anyone with a capacity for reflection on their circumstances, reflection might lead to a more nuanced appreciation of human existence and a sharper quality of inner life. To the extent that any of them, subsequently, lead a life which Victorian reformers would have wished for them, they probably lived their coming days within an elaborated quality of inner life, coping with problems of each day, while memories of a life left behind probably receded into an increasingly distant past.

## 4.4   Ireland

Ireland, even before the Famine, saw a stream of emigrants setting out for urban centers in England, Scotland, and Wales. North America began to attract immigrants in the seventeenth century, and some ventured into the countries of Latin America where Irish family names are encountered today.

For a consideration of Victorian era migrants, young Irish men are less opaque; the Census of Ireland (Jordan, 1998) provides a good deal of social data from which we can sketch an account of how the young men saw themselves and the world around them. The gossoons grew up in a unitary Ireland of four provinces and thirty two counties. Their inner lives were molded by the inherited culture of their families. Ulster's children grew up within the mantle of a fiery Protestantism whose Calvinism was rigid and separatist. On the other hand, the other three provinces Munster, Connacht, and Leinster were Catholic to a large degree, in a synthesis of gaelicism and Roman formality shaped by the Rome-dispatched Archbishop Cullen.

In rural areas the gaelic language persisted prior to the nationalist fervor of later decades. To think about self in gaelic, and to see the world through the medium of that language, structured the young men's mental processes. A language without a clear-cut yes or no suggests a subtlety in the syntax of thinking. The heritage of Hibernian folk tales and ancient laws persisted despite the imposed Anglo-Saxon court system and the conduct of public affairs in English. Irish politicians sought political independence for Queen Victoria's western outpost, or at least home rule— the Irish Parliament having ceded its powers to Westminster as the century began. Daniel O'Connor was the admired figure of the 1840s across Ireland. To the many young men joining the army from Ulster, enlistment affirmed the Britishness of their identity. On the other hand, enlisting was an alternative to a bleak economic future, and a life of stress. A young man's sense of personal worth included a handsome uniform and the regular bugle "call to the cook.house door." However, discipline was harsh, and regret may well have affected many who took the Queen's Shilling.

**Table 4.1** Literacy by Province, 1841, 1851, and 1861[a] as a percentage of the Irish population

| Province | Census year | | |
|---|---|---|---|
| | 1841 | 1851 | 1861 |
| Connacht | 16 | 21 | 28 |
| Munster | 26 | 31 | 40 |
| Ulster | 30 | 35 | 42 |
| Leinster | 34 | 39 | 49 |
| All Ireland | 25 | 33 | 41 |

[a]See the 1861 Census, General Report, Table XIX (Jordan, 1988, Volume 2)

Two writers of the era, Thackery (1869), and Nicholson (1847) described the warmth with which the poor invited them into their squalid dwellings. The young men described in Chap. 3 may have known such charity and capitalized on such memories from childhood. Their sensibilities probably including harsh discipline— long the heritage of nineteenth century Irish families and social institutions such as the law, schooling, and the church in Ireland. A mental resource for the young across Ireland was their increasing literacy. Table 4.1 shows the change across the censuses of 1841, 1851, and 1861 by province.

The youngest army recruits signed up for a long period of service, before the Cardwell reforms of a later decade. They came from a national population which, in 1841, had a mere toehold on literacy, but which grew rapidly as the National Schools system expanded. Educational innovation took hold in Ireland before educational reform in England and Wales. Among the four provinces Connacht in 1841 was mostly illiterate barely surpassing Munster. By 1861 about half of the population was literate, the mechanism being expansion of schooling and the exodus of aging illiterates.

Literacy for the young men accepted by the recruiting sergeants meant several things. Military procedures could be recorded and communicated to the rank and file on paper. Success and failure in military campaigns in remote regions of the world, *e.g.* disasters in Afghanistan, became content for public discussion as newspapers expanded public discourse.

## 4.5   Modernism

As young men embarked on their military service Ireland entered the slow moving process of modernism, one which would increase in pace in a non-linear acceleration. Daniel O'Connell had pursued religious toleration, and had embarked on repeal. In the young men's years a military officer of vision, Thomas Aiskew Larcom entered public life; his impact as a census commissioner was productive, and he also vitalized the justice system. Larcom's actions were a form of modernism, although that term was a twentieth innovation. Another figure whose innovations were an early aspect of modernism in Ireland was the surgeon Dr. William Wilde, father of the playwright, whose innovations improved the visual care available to people.

As reports documented the steady improvement of life in the British Isles, the covert process of mental evolution also began. Young men began to incorporate an implicit secularism into their thinking; they approached authority in several spheres of life with less credulity. Figures in government and church were viewed more critically, and local men ascended in public affairs. To soldiers innovations in military equipment brought modernity in technology into their duties. Medicine began to embrace cleanliness, and Florence Nightingale's innovations spread improving the medical care and welfare of the thin red line. Young men saw a shrinking world, one in which communications expanded, and distant places became familiar.

## 4.6 Elements of Quality of Life

Skills marketable in the economy of Tasmania would have been few, the lads' repertoire having emphasized theft and deception, with violence not out of the picture. However, some skills were in the curriculum at Point Puer, so that imprisonment potentially created marketable skills.

Being juveniles the young convicts were not married. The single state was an advantage when they left Point Puer. It is likely that their commitment to exile in Tasmania came at the end of several sequential convictions ended by an exasperated magistrate. English was the language of all but Gaelic speakers; in general, Tasmania was to be a Protestant bastion, and dispatch of Gaelic speakers from rural Ireland was unlikely. Curiously, among the poor there were elaborate synonyms to hide meaning, terms in an argot impenetrable to the middle classes.

It was unlikely that a juvenile felon would have assets; but street-wise young fellows might well have generated loose cash in ship-board card games. The prior health of the Point Puer lads would have been like that of other young urbanites; that is, short in stature even by the modest standards of the era, and prone to heavy use of tobacco, along with chronic conditions of the limbs and joints. As prospects for employment in the Tasmanian outback they had little strength to offer the lumber industry.

The nearby towns, Hobart Town and Port Arthur, would have appealed to juveniles as sources of pleasure and occasional thieving. The climate of Tasmania was wholesome for ex-urbanites, although cool breezes from the south might have been excessive from time to time. As with other convicts in transit the food on their journey depended for quality on the managers who stocked the ships. Commercial canning was in its infancy as the 1840s opened, and we can hope the young men got enough food of an acceptable quality to sustain them.

Like adult men and women in transit to Australasia junior convicts consulted whichever of the nominally healing disciplines was available. The practical tradition of barber-surgeons brought to bear practical treatment, now two centuries old, whose medications probably were still taken from Nicholas Culpeper' work two centuries later. It seems likely that convict ships were sturdy; less than that standard would have threatened the owners' business plans. The exiled convict who knew of kith and kin in the new world had a supportive system in times of trial, and after completing a sentence. Such support was an item of quality in the life of a young man or woman. Young convicts would have little property beyond what they might carry on their persons. However, after release they might have started on the path to acquire property in the frontier presented by rural Tasmania. To transported felons whose origins lay in Britain's expanding cities the proximity to Hobart Town in Tasmania, and to Sydney on the mainland, suggested an urban settlement congruent with their personal experience. There, one might hear a familiar accent and, indeed, even run into an old acquaintance—an event demonstrating what a small world they might live in. Finally, there were people working under the legal obligations set forth in court endorsed articles of indenture. The best outcome from contracted servitude was discharge and payment in full, and promptly, of what was promised when the articles were registered. Driven by exploitation some servants fled, a fateful step which the law would pursue. Saddest was the situation in which the servant worked faithfully, only to be cheated as the time of service approached its end. Being cheated was a blow to one's sense of justice, and collapsed workers' sense of quality in their lives.

From the accounts of migration from the British Isles to the west, and later to the east it is evident that the series of individual migrations separated by two centuries had elements in common. Both the American migration and that to Australia involved young adults, for the most part. There were dependent children, and there were greybeards leading their family groups. The various hegiras originated in all parts of the United Kingdom. Providing back ground for elements of these great migrations were economic conditions. In the case of the migration to America in the seventeenth century, the British economy was not yet the vital enterprise it would become, beyond mercantilism.

For Australian migrants mentioned here, in particular those whose emigration was voluntary, and in some cases assisted financially, the British economy was slowly expanding, but in doing so it left some people behind. The post-Napoleonic years saw chronic unemployment, and the beginning of a serious decline in work at jobs beginning to shift from croft, cottage and rural slum, to an industrial mode of production. For example, Irish weavers who moved to Bradford in West Yorkshire to work on fine fabrics found their horizons under-cut by factory work. On the other hand, both migrations had similar aspects. Both migrations brought English speakers to the edges of two vast, unexplored continents. Both introduced convicted felons who, in the case of Australia, included juvenile convicts sent to Point Puer; the latter an example of high-minded but under-analyzed social policies.

## 4.7  Comparisons

In both American and Australian emigration, there was an occasion for reflection on the quality of one's past life and on the prospects for the new. While generally not an experience to be savored, voluntary or forced, initiated a process of internal dialogue in which bewilderment might be followed by insight into the self. The dimensions of self were expanded by the experience of encountering the new and the hitherto unknown. The vast oceans offered sights which the urban sensibilities of most immigrants came to grasp; such perceptions evolved thereby increasing the depth of thinking as immigrants strived to assimilate the experiences of people and a wider world.

Although two centuries separated the two groups of immigrants addressed here they shared a thought process still rooted in traditional values. For our generation technology introduces social changes at an alarming rate. The rate of change is swift in our generation, but the migrants of the early nineteenth century shared their predecessors' sense of the changing seasons and the social institutions of property rights and morals. Both groups prized conventionality in the organs of their respective social strata, and deviance was scorned. In both generations the powerful prevailed in social matters at local and national levels, although the early nineteenth century reformers sought with some success to derive their energies from continental sources, *i.e.* use of French lesson plans to power the nascent school systems in England and Ireland. On the other hand social policy addressing criminality changed little across the intervening centuries. Expulsion rather than personal reform of criminals was slow to evolve, and prison reform was a slow process.

Crime itself remained static with property offenses being most common; the woman who stole from Samuel Peps' wife Elizabeth in the Restoration years was little changed as her Victorian descendant followed the earlier example (Williams & Godfrey, 2018) Theft of a shirt in Victoria's day brought down on the miscreant the full weight and majesty of the law. In both centuries theft of clothing was usually a solitary affair and the predilection of females. In the case of such crimes the stirrings of social commentary led to formulating juvenile crime as a separate and distinct social problem. In Ireland, Father Theobald Mathew campaigned against abuse of alcohol, and Daniel O'Connell fought for Catholic emancipation. An emerging modernism suggested that the lives of ordinary people might be on the threshold of vast improvements in their quality of life, if only on a distant shore.

## 4.8 Notes

1. The concept of *self* is by no means self-evident. Shobris (1994) observed,
   *"There is no unitary entity we can call self, I or ego...the illusion of a permanent state of selfhood."* (Shobris, p. 378) With regard to what we are thinking Shobris observed that,
   *"...we subjectively interpret the relatively harmonious function* (of the brain) *as evidence for the existence of a self"* (Shobris, p. 388).
   To some psychological theorists any suffestion of a philosophical dualism within the psychology of mind is anathema. The psychological theorists, J. R. Kantor,

for example, denounced the constructs which were not radically empirical. His Interbehavior rejected mind in psychologial theorizing (Kantor, 1959).

2.   For a grasp of childhood as the 1840s opened in Britain see John Leech's series of sketches Leech (1841). Portraits of Children of the Mobility. *Mobility* is the term used by Leech (an artist renowned for his swift sketches of public events) to differentiate poor children he encountered on London streets from the ranks of the favored (the *Nobility*).

3.   The Latin noun, puer, means boy, and the establishment near Hobart, Point Puer, was intended for juvenile offenders only.

# References

Bailyn, B. (1985). *Voyagers to the west*. New York: Knopf.

Bailyn, B. (2012). The barbarous years. New York: Vintage.

de Charms, R. (1968). *Personal causation*. New York: Academic Press.

Ekirch A. R. (2011). Great Britain's secret convict trade to America. *American Historical Review*, 1285–1291.

Evans, J. (2017). *Emigrants: Why the english sailed to the new world*. London: Weidenfeld and Nicholson.

Holmes, S. (2019). The identity illusion. *New York Review of Books, 66,* 44–48.

Jordan, T. E. (1998). *The Census of Ireland 1821–1911. General reports* (Vol. 3). NY: Mellen.

Kantor, J. (1959). A preface in interbehavioral psychology.

Leech, J. (1841). *Portraits of Children of the Mobility*. London: Bentley.

Maslow, A. (1954). *Motivation and personality*. New York: Harper and Row.

Nicholson, A. (1847). *Ireland's welcome to the stranger*. New York: Baker and Scribner.

Thackery, W. (1869). *The Irish Sketchbook*. London: Smith, Elder.

Wareing, J. (2017). *Indentured migration and the servant trade from London to America 1618–1718: "There is a Great Want of Servants"*. Oxford: Oxford University Press.

Werner, E. (1989). *Vulnerable but invincible: A longitudinal study of resilient children and youth*. Berkely: University of California Press.

Williams, L., & Godfrey, B. (2018). *Criminal women: Researching the lives of female criminals in Britain and Australia*. UK: Pen and Sword.